SpringerBriefs in Computer Science

SpringerBriefs present concise summaries of cutting-edge research and practical applications across a wide spectrum of fields. Featuring compact volumes of 50 to 125 pages, the series covers a range of content from professional to academic.

Typical topics might include:

- A timely report of state-of-the art analytical techniques
- A bridge between new research results, as published in journal articles, and a contextual literature review
- A snapshot of a hot or emerging topic
- An in-depth case study or clinical example
- A presentation of core concepts that students must understand in order to make independent contributions.

Briefs allow authors to present their ideas and readers to absorb them with minimal time investment. Briefs will be published as part of Springer's eBook collection, with millions of users worldwide. In addition, Briefs will be available for individual print and electronic purchase. Briefs are characterized by fast, global electronic dissemination, standard publishing contracts, easy-to-use manuscript preparation and formatting guidelines, and expedited production schedules. We aim for publication 8–12 weeks after acceptance. Both solicited and unsolicited manuscripts are considered for publication in this series.

**Indexing: This series is indexed in Scopus, Ei-Compendex, and zbMATH **

Michael Bouzinier · Dmitry Etin ·
Naeem Khoshnevis · Max Shad · Scott Yockel

Research Data that Can Be Trusted

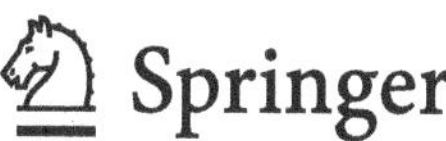

Michael Bouzinier
Harvard University
Cambridge, MA, USA

IDEXX Laboratories
Westbrook, ME, USA

Naeem Khoshnevis
Harvard University
Cambridge, MA, USA

Scott Yockel
Harvard University
Cambridge, MA, USA

Dmitry Etin
Technische Hochschule Deggendorf
Deggendorf, Germany

Max Shad
Harvard University
Cambridge, MA, USA

ISSN 2191-5768 ISSN 2191-5776 (electronic)
SpringerBriefs in Computer Science
ISBN 978-3-032-21031-9 ISBN 978-3-032-21032-6 (eBook)
https://doi.org/10.1007/978-3-032-21032-6

This Springer imprint is published by the registered company Springer Nature Switzerland AG
The registered company address is: Gewerbestrasse 11, 6330 Cham, Switzerland

Preface

This book began with a practical frustration. Working with health data pipelines, we repeatedly encountered situations where understanding what had actually been done to data required archaeology rather than documentation. Scripts accumulated in repositories, transformation logic was scattered across notebooks and team memory and the connection between regulatory requirements and implemented safeguards existed mainly in the heads of those who had built the systems. When personnel changed or projects evolved, this implicit knowledge eroded. Reproducing a dataset meant reverse engineering code. Demonstrating compliance meant assembling narratives after the fact.

This frustration became sharper as our own work moved across contexts. We began with genomic data preparation and the development of tools for interpretation and visualisation in clinical research settings. Over time, the same problems reappeared across broader modalities and larger data environments, where pipelines were built and operated as shared infrastructure rather than as project artefacts. Supporting trusted research environment teams at Harvard, we saw how quickly transformation complexity outpaced the practical ability of any individual to reconstruct what had happened and how brittle trust becomes when it depends on institutional memory.

The frustration deepened as regulatory expectations grew. Instruments such as the AI Act and the European Health Data Space Regulation now ask organisations to explain how datasets were assembled, how biases were addressed and how transformations relate to intended uses. These are reasonable questions. The problem is that most data infrastructures cannot answer them without substantial manual reconstruction. Documentation exists, but it describes systems at a level of abstraction that leaves the interpretive questions unanswered.

We came to see this as more than an engineering inconvenience. Data, especially health data, is often compared to oil, a valuable resource waiting to be extracted. We find a different analogy more apt: health data resembles shale. It is abundant but difficult to access, fragmented across regulatory landscapes, inconsistent in quality and costly to refine into something usable. The techniques required are complex and the provenance of what emerges matters as much as the output itself.

This book is our attempt to address the problem at its root. Rather than proposing better documentation practices or additional compliance layers, we argue for a representational shift: capturing what happens to data as part of how data is processed, in forms that are structured enough to be queried, compared and evaluated. The technical vehicle is a domain-specific language integrated with descriptive workflow tools. The broader aim is an infrastructure in which provenance supports trust rather than merely recording activity.

The book is intended for those who design, operate, regulate or depend on data pipelines in health and research settings. It assumes familiarity with data engineering concepts but does not require expertise in any particular technology. We have tried to write for readers who need to reason about these problems over the coming decades, not merely the current tool cycle.

The General Introduction sets out the argument and structure in full.

Boston, MA, USA
Vienna, Austria
December 2025

Michael Bouzinier
Dmitry Etin

Acknowledgements The authors are grateful to everyone who has made this book possible. Special thanks go to Francesca Dominici, Danielle Braun and Michelle Audirac from the Harvard T. H. Chan School of Public Health, who both provided funding for the engineering effort of developing Dorieh Data Platform and devoted many hours to invaluable discussions about research data platforms and the handling of health data.

We are indebted to Francesco Pontiggia, who was responsible for building the secure infrastructure for Dorieh and who read drafts of this book and provided important comments. We also thank Chigozirim Ben, Daniel Nwosu, Justin Martel, Milson Munakami, Peter Onovakpuri and Matthew Benjamin Sabath from Harvard University Research Computing, who at various times were involved in designing, building and testing Dorieh. Eugenia Lvova from Deggendorf Institute of Technology contributed to the ideation of several sections. Conversations with Michael Bukatin about invariant properties of self-modifying systems inspired the idea of using predicates to validate drifts in evolving AI models.

Finally, we thank Sergey Trifonov, who read one of the earliest drafts of this manuscript and encouraged Michael Bouzinier to proceed with this work.

Competing Interests The authors have no competing interests to declare that are relevant to the content of this manuscript.

Author Contributions

Dmitry Etin and Michael Bouzinier jointly wrote Part I. Michael Bouzinier wrote Parts II and IV, while Dmitry Etin wrote Part III. Scott Yockel supervised the entire project, from the design and development of the Dorieh Data Platform to the writing of the manuscript. Max Shad played an indispensable role in the design and development of Dorieh, while Naeem Khoshnevis contributed to the design and implementation and tested many data-processing workflows. Naeem Khoshnevis also worked on the synthetic data for Medicare claims. All authors read the final manuscript and made valuable suggestions for its improvement.

Contents

About the Authors

Michael Bouzinier is Senior Research Software Engineer within University Research Computing and an AI Data Architect at IDEXX Laboratories. He has over 30 years of diverse experience in software research and development and 10 years as a professional educator. Michael's intellectual interests include semiotics, natural language processing and text analytics, data visualization, evolutionary and medical genetics, computer simulations and explainable AI. Michael is co-founder of Forome, a collaborative initiative advancing open-source and research-driven tooling for transparent and auditable health data pipelines, including structured provenance. Throughout his career, he has worked and led diverse international teams, successfully collaborating with developers and researchers from within the US, UK, Sweden, Finland, Belgium, the Netherlands and Japan.

Over the years Michael has had several publications and has presented at various software development conferences including TheServerSide, Devoxx, QCon, Jazoon, JavaOne, InCoB2010 and ISMB/ECCB 2019, 2022 and 2025.

Publications: https://orcid.org/0000-0002-3161-5601

Dmitry Etin is a health data governance and interoperability advisor working at the intersection of technology, regulation and innovation. He works with health ministries, national digital health authorities, hospital networks and health technology organisations on regulation-ready data architectures, including federated environments for secondary use such as trusted research environments. Dmitry is involved in European initiatives spanning the European Health Data Space, governance for secondary use, and interoperability across regulatory and research contexts. His work also covers medicines interoperability, preparedness and health emergency governance, and Horizon-funded initiatives advancing interoperable EHR systems across the European Union. Together with Michael Bouzinier, Dmitry is co-founder of Forome, a collaborative initiative advancing open-source and research-driven tooling for transparent and auditable health data pipelines, including structured provenance. Earlier in his career, he built and led an IT department in a hospital setting and later worked with organisations including Tieto, Dell and Oracle on large-scale interoperability programmes. Dmitry lectures at Deggendorf Institute of Technology and holds an M.Sc. in Computer Science.

Contact: dmitry.etin@forome.org; LinkedIn: https://www.linkedin.com/in/dmitryetin/

Naeem Khoshnevis is a Research Software Engineer within University Research Computing. In this role, Naeem designs, builds and optimizes software applications for researchers across Harvard University. Naeem has a superior mathematical and numerical analysis background and has developed, documented, debugged, extended and refactored numerous scientific software applications for research groups, helping them successfully carry out their projects. Before joining University Research Computing, Naeem conducted research on large-scale ground motion simulations. Having an interdisciplinary educational background in Engineering, Applied Science and Computer Science, he values the importance of good software engineering practices in reliable and reproducible scientific research. In his free time, Naeem enjoys reading, running, cooking and watching documentaries.

https://rc.harvard.edu/about-us/naeem-khoshnevis/

Max Shad is Senior Director of AI/ML Research Engineering at the Kempner Institute for the Study of Natural and Artificial Intelligence at Harvard University. In this role, he leads the computational program of the Kempner Institute, ensuring the provision of advanced Research Computing (RC) tools/services and expert Research Engineering support. He works to leverage High-Performance Computing (HPC), particularly in Machine Learning (ML) and AI research, to facilitate pioneering discoveries in AI, ML and computational biology. In addition, his role at the Kempner Institute involves strategic planning for AI HPC cluster compute/storage hardware and networking, collaborating closely with teams at the Faculty of Arts and Sciences Research Computing (FASRC) at Harvard and the Massachusetts Green High-Performance Computing Center (MGHPCC).

Prior to his current position, Max served as Director of Engineering and Associate Director for Research Software Engineering at Harvard, where he led the establishment of Harvard's first RSE team. His work has significantly advanced RSE, focusing on designing, building and maintaining research software and data services in various domains (neuroscience, life sciences, medical sciences, engineering, computer science, applied math, astrophysics, business, public health and design). With a Ph.D. in Mechanical Engineering (focusing on computational science and HPC) and a graduate certificate in Data Science and ML from Harvard, his research interests include AI/ML, complex fluids, HPC and innovative big data analytics. As an active member of the RSE and HPC communities, Max has chaired several conferences and initiated the New England RSE regional group, advocating for idea exchange and collaboration among local RSE groups. Max is Member of the Research Computing and Data (RCD) Council at Harvard University.

https://scholar.harvard.edu/mmsh/home

Scott Yockel is the University Research Computing Officer at Harvard. In this role, Scott works with researchers across campus to develop and champion a university-wide research computing strategy in support of Harvard's research mission. Scott is focused on identifying emerging needs, engaging with faculty, school, and university leadership to articulate those needs, and identifying possible solutions and funding mechanisms. He is spearheading the implementation of these initiatives and articulating their success with concrete measures, as well as developing plans for the long-term sustainability of research computing at Harvard. Over the last several years, Scott has been deeply involved in national and regional efforts such as CaRCC and MGHPCC. In this newly expanded role, he will be more deeply engaged in these efforts that increasingly involve national-level cyberinfrastructure resources and the development and professionalization of research computing staff. For example, he is PI/co-PI on a number of externally funded projects, including the New England Research Cloud, Northeast Storage Exchange and the NSF Center of Excellence, RCD-Nexus.

https://rc.harvard.edu/about-us/scott-yockel/

Chapter 1
Introduction

Modern healthcare and health research increasingly depend on complex data pipelines that assemble, curate and transform heterogeneous sources such as clinical records, diagnostic data, claims and registries. These pipelines are the practical means by which secondary use of health data becomes possible, because most datasets that support research, policy and decision support are not collected as such but are produced through successive refinements that reconcile formats, units, coding systems, time bases and inclusion criteria. At the same time, regulation, institutional governance and professional standards increasingly require not only that data be handled securely but that organisations can explain how datasets were assembled, transformed and validated across their lifecycle and they do so in ways that assume a level of insight into data preparation that document-centric practices cannot reliably provide.

This book centers on preserving provenance within data preparation workflows and proposes best practices for doing so. But before introducing technical mechanisms, it is prudent to ask why data preparation remains a central concern at all. Given the capabilities of modern data science and artificial intelligence, it is tempting to assume that raw data can simply be fed into analytical systems and refined later by modelling techniques, yet in health settings this assumption fails in ways that are costly, difficult to detect and, once embedded in downstream results, difficult to correct.

From "Data Is the New Oil" to Real Value

Is Data the New Oil, as The Economist famously suggested on its cover in 2017? The short answer is no, because raw data must be refined to be useful. The popular comparison of data to oil captures the idea of latent value, but it underplays the difficulty of producing reusable health datasets. A different analogy is often more

M. Bouzinier et al., *Research Data that Can Be Trusted*,
SpringerBriefs in Computer Science, https://doi.org/10.1007/978-3-032-21032-6_1

accurate: health data resembles shale. It is abundant but difficult to access, fragmented across institutional and regulatory landscapes, inconsistent in quality and costly to refine into something usable. The techniques required are complex and the provenance of what emerges matters as much as the output itself, because refinement choices shape what the dataset can legitimately support.

Let us consider how value is derived from data, especially through secondary use, when new knowledge or utility is produced beyond the original purpose of collection. In healthcare, this means understanding the journey from primary data sources to societal benefit. Value for secondary use of health data emerges when a new purpose is defined and the data are altered accordingly, when new knowledge is extracted beyond the primary purpose and when the full journey from sources to outcomes can be traced and understood.

Data to Value Workflow

This value generally materialises through two distinct pathways: research and policy and decision support systems. These pathways create societal benefits in different but complementary ways. Research and policy shape population-level decisions, while decision support systems influence real-time, individual-level care and operations. Figure 1.1 illustrates how data flow when these two pathways are at work.

Both pathways begin with depositing raw data into an analytics-optimised repository, typically a data warehouse or an equivalent curated layer. From there, the same underlying data can travel along two distinct routes. On one route, researchers use warehouse data to build statistical models, conduct epidemiological and health

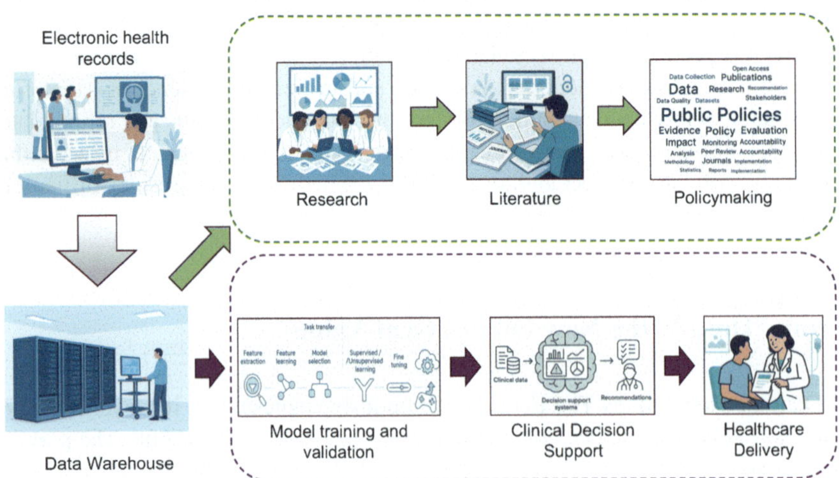

Fig. 1.1 Data to value workflow

services studies and generate evidence that informs guidelines, reimbursement models and public health policy. On the other route, the same data are used to train machine learning and AI models that power clinical decision support, risk prediction and operational optimisation, producing outputs that may be acted upon in care delivery and health system operations. Together, these pathways describe how secondary use of health data is translated into societal benefit.

Pattern Detection and Data Preparation

Both research analysis and model training can be understood as forms of pattern detection, recognising or learning regularities in the data. Humans are remarkably good at this, and modern systems extend this capacity through statistical learning and machine learning. However, the quality of patterns detected depends fundamentally on the quality of the input data and the quality of input data in practice is not a property of the source systems alone but a property of the transformations applied during preparation.

This is the point at which the work of data engineering becomes visible. Data engineers do not simply move data between systems, they make a sequence of decisions that render data computable and comparable, reconciling incompatible encodings, aligning time windows, removing duplicates, defining cohorts, imputing or excluding values, constructing derived variables, masking or aggregating sensitive fields and applying validation rules that determine what is accepted as plausible. These steps are often necessary, but they are also interpretive, because they embed assumptions about meaning, quality and fitness for purpose.

Figure 1.2 illustrates the challenge: on the right; a clean pattern is easily detected, in the middle it is hidden by cloudiness; and on the left it is obscured even further by dirty inputs.

More critically, poor preparation does not only make patterns harder to detect, it can produce bad knowledge. Humans and algorithms alike may infer spurious, non-existent patterns from corrupted data, or may fail to detect genuine structure that is

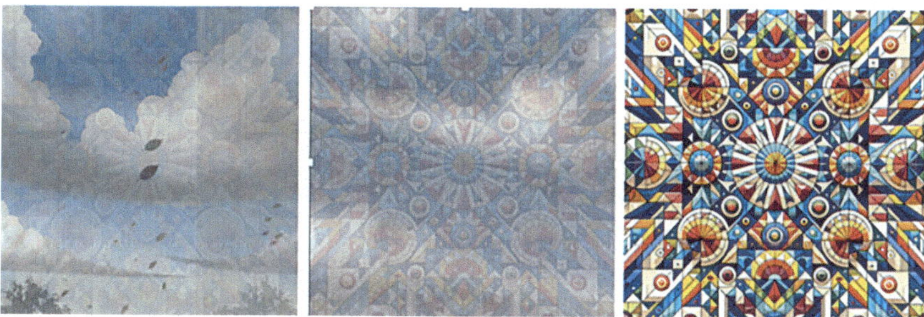

Fig. 1.2 Buried signals: revealing patterns in dirty data

present but obscured. To avoid erroneous conclusions and inflated costs, rigorous data preparation becomes essential, including steps such as normalisation, harmonisation and data cleansing.

Mad Hatter's Data Preparation Parable

Recall the exercises from elementary school to fill the missing number, a process rooted in pattern detection. Imagine the Mad Hatter recording air temperatures over time. The true values follow the Fibonacci sequence, each value from the third onward is the sum of the prior two and the missing value should be straightforward to infer.

However, when data collection is delegated, the results are not ideal. March Hare's data jumbles text with numerals, obscuring the pattern until uniform representation is imposed through normalisation. Cheshire Cat's data mixes units, Celsius, Kelvin and Fahrenheit, where the values are correct in context but only become interpretable as a sequence after harmonisation to a common unit. White Rabbit's data omits or distorts numbers, illustrating why cleansing can be decisive, because it can conceal true structure or introduce artefacts that invite entirely wrong inferences. Table 1.1 summarises the illustration.

This parable is intentionally simple, but it captures what becomes consequential in real pipelines. Preparation is not a decorative step; it is the mechanism that makes pattern detection possible and makes downstream interpretation defensible. Normalisation and harmonisation are often reversible in the sense that they preserve a one to one mapping between input and output. Cleansing may delete, substitute, impute, mask, or otherwise alter values, changing the evidentiary basis of downstream analyses and models and potentially reshaping representation across groups, which is precisely why these choices require traceability rather than implicit acceptance.

Table 1.1 Mad Hatter's data preparation

1	2	3	4	5	6	7	8	9	10	Observation
1	2	3	5	8	13	21	34	55	?	Ideal data
One	2	3	Five	8	$0.13*10^2$	Twenty One	Thirty Four	55	?	Data requires normalization
274.15	2.0	3.0	278.15	46.4	13	69.8	307.5	55.0	?	Data requires harmonization
1		3	4	9	15	25	36	51	?	Data requires cleansing

Data Warehouses and Feature Stores

To manage these transformation challenges at scale, organisations rely on specialised infrastructure such as data warehouses and feature stores. A data warehouse provides normalised, harmonised and cleansed data to end-users, including researchers and model builders. A feature store builds on this foundation, becoming a centralised system for managing machine learning features, acting as a single source of truth to store, share, discover and serve consistent data.

Yet neither a warehouse nor a feature store is trustworthy merely because it exists. Trust depends on whether it is possible to determine what the repository contains, why it contains it in that form and how that form was produced. A data dictionary helps establish shared meaning at the level of variables and representations. Provenance provides the record of transformations that produced the published outputs. The core point is not that every transformation must be exhaustively explained in prose, but that the record of what happened must be sufficiently structured that reconstruction is not the default mode of assurance.

Data Preparation in Research Workflows

Trustworthy, well documented data are essential for scientific research, where findings must be independently validated and where errors can propagate through multiple downstream analyses. Historically, data were often small enough that manual tracking and improvisation could suffice to make work explainable and validatable by peers. Modern secondary use involves larger datasets, more reuse, more heterogeneity and more automation, and it carries higher risks, including in settings involving personally identifiable and protected health information. As data are used for downstream model training, the stakes for accuracy, transparency and accountability rise, with real-world consequences in policy and care.

This is also where reproducibility meets oversight. Reproducing a result is rarely a matter of re-running a model alone; it is a matter of reconstituting the dataset as it existed at a specific time under a specific set of transformations and of demonstrating that the dataset was produced under constraints consistent with the declared purpose. When preparation steps remain scattered across scripts, notebooks and tacit conventions, reproducibility becomes a reconstruction exercise, and oversight becomes an interpretive narrative assembled after the fact.

At the same time, external expectations around traceability and justification have widened. Regulation, institutional governance and professional standards increasingly ask organisations to explain how datasets were assembled, how quality and bias risks were addressed and how transformations relate to intended uses and permitted purposes. The challenge is that most infrastructures cannot answer these questions without substantial manual reconstruction. Documentation exists, but it often describes systems at a level of abstraction that leaves interpretive questions unanswered, while executable scripts remain difficult to read as evidence.

Problem and Motivation

The book starts from the observation that this is a structural rather than an administrative difficulty. As data processing workflows grow in complexity and expectations proliferate, the volume and granularity of evidentiary material needed for informed review exceeds what human-bounded mechanisms can absorb. Under these conditions, producing more narrative artefacts risks drifting toward formality checks rather than substantive understanding, because the limiting factor becomes the ability to reconstruct what happened, not the willingness to report.

Conceptual Architecture

The argument is developed within an architecture of trust for data-intensive health systems. Operational trust concerns secure and predictable environments. Epistemic trust concerns the validity of results. Interpretive trust concerns the transparency of data processes, including whether it is possible to understand how data have been shaped and whether that shaping is appropriate for a given use. The interpretive dimension is often the most fragile, because it requires a bridge between what was executed in code and what must be understood for reproducibility, quality management and accountable reuse.

Between human readable documents and machine executable scripts, a stable representational layer is often missing, one that captures what was actually done to data in terms that can be related to scientific and governance expectations. The central claim of this book is that provenance must be treated as that layer, not merely as a log of activity, and that it must operate at the level of transformations, with semantics that support inspection, comparison and evaluation.

Technical Realisation

On this basis, the book develops a provenance-aware approach to data processing in which transformation history is captured as part of normal operation rather than reconstructed after the fact. The technical contributions are introduced in Part I and developed through Parts II and IV, including a concrete platform implementation used to illustrate how transformation-level provenance, lineage and validation records can be produced consistently within real pipelines and then used as evidence for reproducibility and for recurring interpretive checks.

Applications and Impact

The framework is illustrated on healthcare claims data, where provenance-aware workflows reveal inconsistencies and quality issues that conventional approaches leave implicit. The emphasis is not on producing more documentation, but on making transformations inspectable in a structured form so that reproducibility and accountable reuse can be supported without relying on institutional memory.

Structure of the Book and Intended Audience

The book moves from technical need to conceptual architecture and then returns to implementation foundations. Part I establishes the engineering case for complete provenance and introduces the workflow and language concepts used in the remainder of the book. Part II demonstrates implementation through the Dorieh Data Platform and its application to synthetic and real healthcare claims data. Part III situates these contributions within a broader architecture of trust, analysing the structural limits of current oversight and introducing external predicates over provenance as a form of computable, yet governed, assurance. Part IV provides a classification of transformations and validation operators as a semantic foundation for provenance-aware systems.

Throughout, provenance and compliance-as-code are treated not as ends in themselves but as instruments for sustaining trust in data-intensive health systems at a scale and tempo compatible with contemporary infrastructures, and the argument is developed in a form intended to remain useful over the coming decades rather than the next technology cycle.

Part I
The Need, the Opportunity and the Solution

Chapter 2
The Need for Complete Data Provenance

This chapter explains why complete data provenance is increasingly necessary for secondary use of health data and why traditional approaches do not scale. In modern pipelines, decisive choices are not only which sources were used, but how data were normalised, linked, filtered, imputed, aggregated, suppressed and validated. These steps shape what downstream analyses and models can legitimately claim, yet they are usually recorded as scattered code, partial logs or after-the-fact narratives. We define complete provenance as provenance that is captured automatically during execution, structured for query and comparison, and granular enough to explain how specific outputs were produced. The chapter argues that workflow automation is the practical lever: once workflow topology and transformation operators are explicit, provenance becomes a routine by-product rather than an archaeological reconstruction.

After completing this chapter, readers should be able to:

- Explain why privacy constraints shift reproducibility from artefact sharing to process evidence
- Define complete provenance and distinguish it from logs and dataset-level lineage
- Describe how workflow automation enables automatic capture of transformation-level provenance.

The Challenge of Data Ingestion in Research Workflows

Reproducibility is the ability to replicate results using the same data and methods. In practice, it begins earlier than model training or statistical analysis because it depends on data ingestion workflows that acquire, harmonise and cleanse data from continuously updated public and proprietary sources, and that turn operational records into research-ready datasets.

Reproducibility and repeatability are central in computational science. When source data change, acquisition and preparation workflows must be rerun. These

M. Bouzinier et al., *Research Data that Can Be Trusted*,
SpringerBriefs in Computer Science, https://doi.org/10.1007/978-3-032-21032-6_2

workflows are often described in standard operating procedures (SOPs) that assume manual steps, which are time-consuming and, more importantly, error-prone—making a strong case for automation. However, automation alone does not guarantee reproducibility. Re-execution depends on consistent, fully specified dependencies and configuration, typically achieved through containerised runtimes and pinned package versions, rather than identical hardware, if results are to remain comparable across reruns.

Domain experts are primarily responsible for formulating questions, defining cohorts, designing analyses and interpreting results, not for engineering data infrastructure. Yet they must work across disconnected systems, fragmented tools and heterogeneous data sources, and often trust underlying technology stacks they did not design and cannot easily inspect. In healthcare and other regulated domains, privacy, security and compliance restrictions frequently prevent raw data from being published or shared, so the common remedy of "share data and code" is not viable: sharing code alone does not reproduce the controlled environment around the data. Reproducibility and audit therefore become problems of process replication rather than artefact distribution. This forces subject-matter experts to navigate complex technical and governance constraints simultaneously, slowing iteration and complicating quality assurance, while investment by research funders and independent software vendors in robust end-to-end workflow tooling remains limited.

External researchers must be able to replicate workflows in their own environment, often under different hardware and regulatory requirements. When confidential healthcare data cannot move, a practical approach is to share infrastructure patterns rather than datasets, allowing institutions to reproduce results on their own data under their own agreements. Infrastructure as Code (IaC), combined with appropriate containerised environments and configuration management, supports standardised and compliant execution environments during data processing.

Researchers note that providing enough detail for full reproducibility is hard in computational science (Ball 2023), and reproducibility checklists for published research have been suggested and widely discussed (Pineau et al. 2021). As observed by Raff, only 63.5% of 255 papers using AI methods could be reproduced as reported, while reproducibility rises to 85% if the original authors help by actively supplying data and code (Pineau et al. 2021; Raff 2019). Ball cites Joseph Cohen, a scientist at Amazon AWS Health AI, who notes that "If there aren't enough public data sets, then researchers can't evaluate their models correctly and end up publishing low-quality results that show great performance" (Ball 2023). In health-related research, public datasets are often unavailable, and data containing personally identifiable information (PII) or protected health information (PHI) are subject to strict compliance regimes. This makes reproducible ingestion and preparation workflows especially important, because different teams must be able to feed restricted datasets into analytical and modelling pipelines in comparable ways without exchanging the raw data itself.

Data quality adds a further constraint, especially when research involves AI. Experiences during the COVID-19 pandemic illustrate how easily models can exploit artefacts that correlate with labels but are not clinically meaningful. As Ball notes, one study of chest X-ray images initially reported success in identifying COVID-19 cases, yet closer examination revealed that the model could still identify cases using blank background sections of the images, indicating that it had detected consistent differences in background rather than clinically relevant features (Ball 2023).

Even with standardised execution environments and repeatable orchestration, a gap remains. Teams can rerun a workflow, but they often cannot explain what was done to the data at the level needed to reproduce a dataset as an evidence object. To make reruns interpretable, the steps that reshape data must be captured during execution, at the level of concrete transformations and their parameters, rather than inferred later from scripts and team memory.

Challenges in Data Governance and Compliance

Reproducibility and provenance are critical to any good science, but the stakes are dramatically higher when research involves personally identifiable or otherwise sensitive health data, where the risk of adverse consequences is greater for both individuals and institutions. As healthcare relies more heavily on data-driven systems and decisions, some degree of government regulation of data use is unavoidable: safeguards for privacy, security and ethics have to keep pace with these developments. At the same time, organisations face increasingly detailed expectations about how data must be governed. They are expected to show not only that data are handled securely, but also that data quality, privacy safeguards and traceability can be demonstrated in a form suitable for independent review.

In Europe, for example, the European AI Act classifies certain AI systems, including those in healthcare, as high-risk and imposes documentation, risk management and transparency requirements. The practical implication is that organisations must be able to account for how training and evaluation data were prepared and why those choices are appropriate for the intended use, not only where data came from or which tools were used. As frameworks evolve, teams often struggle to align day-to-day pipeline operations with the kinds of evidence these requirements presuppose.

In this setting, provenance is not merely an internal engineering convenience. When captured automatically and in structured form, it becomes the bridge between operational data processing and governance obligations for transparency, reproducibility and traceability, without relying on bespoke narrative reconstruction each time evidence is needed.

A further complication is that compliance is rarely one-dimensional. Obligations differ across jurisdictions and institutional contexts, and they overlap in ways that increase operational burden. This book therefore treats provenance not only as a record of activity, but as an operational layer for managing diverse expectations through consistent, reusable evidence, and for reducing reliance on document-centric compliance practices that strain at scale.

Challenges in Data Quality and Reproducibility

Data quality is a cornerstone of both scientific integrity and regulatory compliance. In healthcare and AI workflows, persistent obstacles to achieving and maintaining data quality tend to accumulate across multi-stage pipelines, so small inconsistencies early in ingestion can become material distortions downstream.

Fragmentation and silos are a first-order difficulty. Healthcare data often reside in disparate systems, from hospital electronic health records (EHRs) and departmental lab or radiology systems to insurance claims and specialised research databases such as disease registries. The same patient's admission, laboratory results and follow-up visit may be stored under different identifiers and schemas in each of these systems, with no reliable way to link them. These silos create inconsistencies, gaps and duplication, making consolidation for analysis and reporting difficult and often brittle.

A second difficulty is lack of standardisation. Data formats, terminologies and quality conventions vary across institutions and jurisdictions, and the mismatch is frequently semantic rather than cosmetic. Common classes of discrepancy include geographic identifiers, where administrative codes and statistical tabulations follow different definitions, for example:

- USPS ZIP codes versus Census Bureau ZIP Code Tabulation Areas (ZCTA), where the cross-mapping can shift across years.
- Units of measurement, where metric and Imperial conventions are mixed and temperatures may be recorded in Kelvin, Fahrenheit, or Celsius.
- Demographic coding, including race and ethnicity, where specifications such as Transformed Medicaid Statistical Information System (T-MSIS) and Research Triangle Institute (RTI) conflict.
- Diagnostic coding, where reliance on International Classification of Diseases (ICD) is complicated by structural changes across major versions, such as ICD-9 to ICD-10.
- Specialised ontologies such as Human Phenotype Ontology (HPO), and clinical data structures, where standards and models such as HL7 v2, Fast Healthcare Interoperability Resources (FHIR), Clinical Document Architecture (CDA) and Observational Medical Outcomes Partnership (OMOP) Common Data Model impose different representations that must be reconciled.

Taken together, these issues contribute to what is often described as a reproducibility crisis in data-intensive science. Even when workflows are documented, results can diverge due to differences in preprocessing choices, software environments and human interpretation of ambiguous cases, particularly when disambiguation rules and data cleaning heuristics are embedded in code rather than expressed explicitly (Tang and Borlak 2024).

The consequences are pronounced in AI systems, where training data quality directly shapes model behaviour. Biases and artefacts introduced during preparation can propagate into models and lead to outcomes that are inaccurate or discriminatory.

This is also why high-risk AI governance regimes emphasise dataset quality management and transparency about training, testing and validation data, expectations that are difficult to satisfy without structured records of how data were prepared.

Accountability and Ethical Concerns

Accountability and ethics are central to the discourse on data governance (United Nations 2024). As AI systems increasingly influence clinical and administrative decisions, failures are not confined to technical performance. They can translate into denial of services, delayed treatment, inequitable outcomes and loss of trust. The class-action lawsuit alleging that UnitedHealth used the "nH Predict" algorithm to deny medically necessary post-acute care for Medicare Advantage patients illustrates how opaque automated decision-making can be contested when its impacts are material and difficult to justify.

The integration of AI into clinical workflows has triggered an active public discussion regarding a potential crisis of transparency. Reporting from The New York Times and The Wall Street Journal has highlighted that many FDA-cleared AI tools provide limited visibility into training data and validation conditions. When such context is unavailable, clinicians and reviewers cannot judge whether a system's reported performance is transferable to their population or setting. Black-box systems can be susceptible to "adversarial attacks", where data are manipulated to trick the system.

These concerns connect directly to the evidentiary limits described earlier. Traditional validation approaches prioritise performance metrics, yet accountability requires the ability to explain how data were prepared, which assumptions were applied and how changes in data or context might alter behaviour. Without this, oversight risks becoming a debate about outcomes without a shared account of the processes that produced them. Provenance therefore matters here not as a retrospective narrative but as a routine, structured record of data work that can support justification, review and improvement.

In the next chapter, we turn to workflow automation and domain-specific languages as the technical foundation for implementing comprehensive provenance in healthcare and AI systems.

References

Ball, P. (2023). Is AI leading to a reproducibility crisis in science? *Nature, 624*(7990), 22–25. https://doi.org/10.1038/d41586-023-03817-6

Pineau, J., Vincent-Lamarre, P., Sinha, K., Larivière, V., Beygelzimer, A., d'Alché-Buc, F., Fox, E., & Larochelle, H. (2021). Improving reproducibility in machine learning research (a report from the NeurIPS 2019 reproducibility program). *The Journal of Machine Learning Research, 22*(1), 164:7459–164:7478.

Raff, E. (2019). *A Step Toward Quantifying Independently Reproducible Machine Learning Research* (No. arXiv:1909.06674). arXiv. https://doi.org/10.48550/arXiv.1909.06674

Tang, S., & Borlak, J. (2024). Genomics of human NAFLD: Lack of data reproducibility and high interpatient variability in drug target expression as major causes of drug failures. *Hepatology (Baltimore, Md.)*, *80*(4), 901–915. https://doi.org/10.1097/HEP.0000000000000780

United Nations. (2024). *Governing AI for Humanity*. United Nations.

Chapter 3
The Opportunity: Advancement of Workflow Automation

Having established the practical challenges of healthcare data handling in Chap. 2, we now turn to the technological landscape. To appreciate the solution proposed in Chap. 4, we must first understand the tools currently available for expressing and executing pipelines. This chapter traces the evolution of workflow automation, moving from general-purpose procedural code to frameworks that make pipeline topology explicit. We examine the progression from API-based data processing frameworks, such as Apache Spark and Hadoop, and from orchestrators, such as Apache Airflow, toward descriptive workflow languages such as Snakemake and Common Workflow Language (CWL). By separating pipeline structure from the implementation of individual steps, these languages improve portability and repeatability, and they make it possible to derive workflow-level lineage graphs directly from the declared topology.

After completing this chapter, readers should be able to:

1. Compare procedural, API-based and descriptive workflow automation approaches
2. Explain how descriptive workflow languages achieve portability and repeatability
3. Describe how declared pipeline topology enables derivation of workflow-level lineage graphs.

Current Approaches to Workflow Automation

An integral part of any data warehouse are the data acquisition workflows, typically represented by Extract Transform Load (ETL) or Extract Load Transform (ELT) pipelines. These data acquisition and processing pipelines are best based on the traditional dataflow programming paradigm (Schwarzkopf 2020). For most computational studies, their data acquisition workflow can be represented as a data processing

M. Bouzinier et al., *Research Data that Can Be Trusted*,
SpringerBriefs in Computer Science, https://doi.org/10.1007/978-3-032-21032-6_3

pipeline. This pipeline consists of steps, each being either a script, a binary executable, or a specific data transformation within a data warehouse.

Some steps are dependent on the results of others, which allows every workflow to be represented as a Directed Acyclic Graph (DAG), as illustrated in Fig. 3.1. In this example DAG, nodes correspond to specific tasks such as **Ingest** yearly enrollment or admissions files, **Harmonize** their schemas, **Consolidate** Enrollments/ Admissions across years and build the **Master Beneficiaries Index**. Edges encode the dependencies between these tasks: for instance, each **Harmonize** node can only run after its corresponding **Ingest** step has completed; **Consolidate Enrollments** depends on all three yearly harmonization steps; **Cleanse Admissions** depends on both the consolidated admissions data and the **Master Beneficiaries Index** and **Build Enrollments Table** nodes to enforce referential integrity. Finally, the gold-layer QC node (Admissions QC Metrics) can only execute after the admissions table is built.

Historically, people have moved from expressing the data processing logic in universal procedural programming languages to dedicated API- and command-based workflow definition frameworks and finally introduced specialized workflow definition languages. In the following paragraphs, we will briefly review these approaches. An extensive review of legacy approaches to define a data processing pipeline is available (Leipzig 2017).

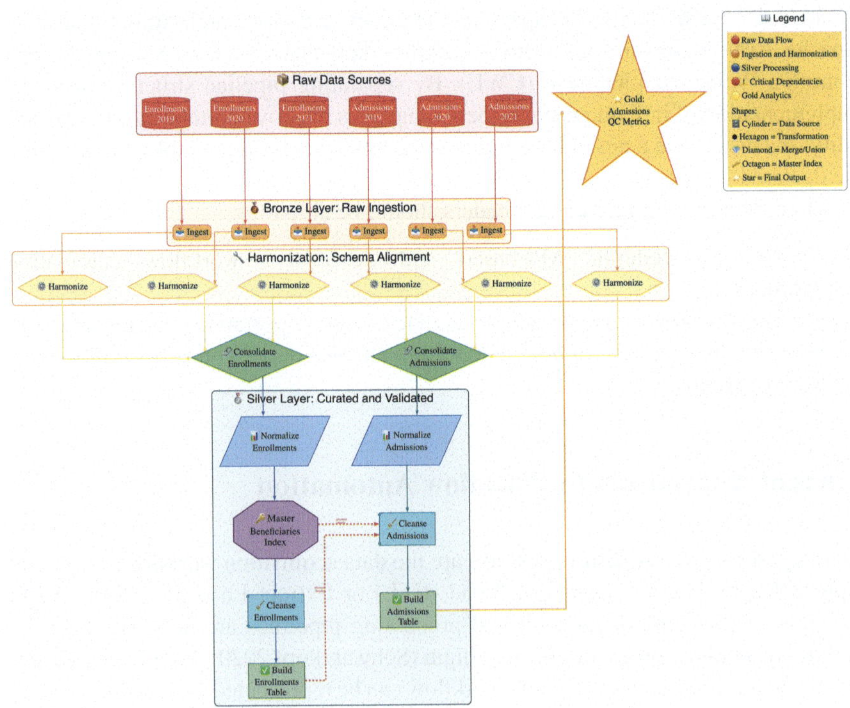

Fig. 3.1 Sample DAG for building feature store for US medicare claims data

Procedural Languages

The majority of widely used programming languages fall into this category, which includes C/C++, Python and Java. They are based on the concept of "procedure calls", which means they follow a step-by-step approach. They solve a problem by breaking it down into a collection of variables, routines, or subroutines. As universal programming languages, they are capable of expressing a wide range of concepts, including workflow compositions and pipeline logic.

However, this often results in convoluted programs that are economically ineffective to maintain due to the complexity of pipeline topologies, which provide for massive parallelization and multiple dependencies.

API-Based Workflow Definition Frameworks

A step forward from expressing pipeline logic in a conventional programming language is the utilization of API-based frameworks like Apache Spark (Zaharia et al. n.d.) and Apache Hadoop (HDFS Architecture Guide n.d.). This approach requires specific programming for each step. While it enforces good and clean architecture and is efficient in utilizing computational resources, porting legacy pipelines would require a full rewrite. If any tool used in the existing pipeline cannot be programmatically called from within the chosen framework, resolving this issue could be extremely challenging.

Command-Based Workflow Definition Frameworks

These frameworks focus on describing the pipeline topology and can leverage any tool that can be launched from a command line, which makes them well-suited to support incremental porting of legacy pipelines. Examples of command-based frameworks include Apache Airflow (What Is Airflow™?—Airflow Documentation n.d.), Luigi (How To Build a Data Processing Pipeline Using Luigi in Python on Ubuntu 20.04 | DigitalOcean n.d.) and the retired Apache Taverna (Wolstencroft et al. 2013). However, these tools do not explicitly define the inputs, resources and outputs of a pipeline. Thus, these frameworks may not detect when a hardcoded path to a file or a local resource is accidentally used in the workflow.

Descriptive Workflow Languages

Descriptive workflow languages have taken command-based workflow definition frameworks to the next level of automation readiness and portability. These languages include Snakemake (Mölder et al. 2021), Common Workflow Language (CWL) (Methods Included—Communications of the ACM 2022), Workflow Definition Language (WDL) and Nextflow (Di Tommaso et al. 2017) fully address repeatability and reproducibility of data processing pipelines (Ahmed et al. 2021). They focus on the explicit definition of pipeline topology and separate the definition of topology, inputs, requirements and outputs of a workflow from the actual processing algorithms. Most of these languages combine elements of descriptive languages, which focus on the "what" rather than the "how", with elements of functional programming languages that handle data as immutable data streams. The descriptiveness of these languages is demonstrated by their diverse implementations on different platforms. For instance, CWL implementations include Toil (Vivian et al. 2017) and Arvados (The Arvados Authors et al. 2024) which translate CWL documents into commands for various scheduling systems, including Slurm, Amazon Web Services (AWS) Batch and Google Cloud Platform (GCP) Batch. On the other hand, CWL-Airflow (Kotliar et al. 2019), translates CWL documents into Python code for Apache Airflow. Despite these different implementations and platforms, you can reasonably expect to achieve the same results when executing the same CWL workflow.

Descriptive workflow languages were pioneered by the bioinformatics community, where they have since become the standard for complex analysis tasks. However, they have yet to gain a strong foothold in general data science. Examining the reasons behind this siloed success, we argue that the isolation is not due to a lack of utility, but rather specific missing features. By addressing these gaps with the extensions proposed in this book, we believe these languages can be successfully adapted to serve the broader needs of data preparation and provenance, including settings where compliance expectations apply.

Command-based workflow definition frameworks and especially descriptive workflow languages have revolutionized the automation of computational workflows. Importantly, they have also paved a path to documenting dataset-level lineage in downstream analysis by visualizing it as data lineage graphs, depicting the sources of original data and the steps in the data processing workflow that have been performed to build a downstream dataset.

In the realm of dataflow programming, descriptive workflow languages excel in illustrating the data flow necessary for processing, providing a robust framework for defining the edges of a DAG representing a workflow. Yet, these languages remain agnostic regarding the DAG's nodes, which serve as the operators applying data transformations. In line with the dataflow programming paradigm, these operators are treated as 'black boxes' characterized by their defined inputs and outputs.

References

Ahmed, A. E., Allen, J. M., Bhat, T., Burra, P., Fliege, C. E., Hart, S. N., Heldenbrand, J. R., Hudson, M. E., Istanto, D. D., Kalmbach, M. T., Kapraun, G. D., Kendig, K. I., Kendzior, M. C., Klee, E. W., Mattson, N., Ross, C. A., Sharif, S. M., Venkatakrishnan, R., Fadlelmola, F. M., & Mainzer, L. S. (2021). Design considerations for workflow management systems use in production genomics research and the clinic. *Scientific Reports, 11,* 21680. https://doi.org/10.1038/s41598-021-99288-8

Di Tommaso, P., Chatzou, M., Floden, E. W., Barja, P. P., Palumbo, E., & Notredame, C. (2017). Nextflow enables reproducible computational workflows. *Nature Biotechnology, 35*(4), 316–319. https://doi.org/10.1038/nbt.3820

HDFS Architecture Guide. (n.d.). Retrieved December 16, 2025, from https://hadoop.apache.org/docs/r1.2.1/hdfs_design.html

How To Build a Data Processing Pipeline Using Luigi in Python on Ubuntu 20.04 | DigitalOcean. (n.d.). Retrieved February 23, 2024, from https://www.digitalocean.com/community/tutorials/how-to-build-a-data-processing-pipeline-using-luigi-in-python-on-ubuntu-20-04

Kotliar, M., Kartashov, A. V., & Barski, A. (2019). CWL-Airflow: A lightweight pipeline manager supporting Common Workflow Language. *GigaScience, 8*(7), giz084. https://doi.org/10.1093/gigascience/giz084

Leipzig, J. (2017). A review of bioinformatic pipeline frameworks. *Briefings in Bioinformatics, 18*(3), 530–536. https://doi.org/10.1093/bib/bbw020

Methods Included – Communications of the ACM. (2022, June 1). https://cacm.acm.org/research/methods-included/

Mölder, F., Jablonski, K. P., Letcher, B., Hall, M. B., Tomkins-Tinch, C. H., Sochat, V., Forster, J., Lee, S., Twardziok, S. O., Kanitz, A., Wilm, A., Holtgrewe, M., Rahmann, S., Nahnsen, S., & Köster, J. (2021). *Sustainable data analysis with Snakemake* (No. 10:33). F1000Research. https://doi.org/10.12688/f1000research.29032.2

Schwarzkopf, M. (2020, March 7). *The Remarkable Utility of Dataflow Computing – ACM SIGOPS.* https://www.sigops.org/2020/the-remarkable-utility-of-dataflow-computing/

The Arvados Authors, Amstutz, P., César, N., Clegg, T., Di Pentima, L., Kutyła, D., Li, J., Smith, S., Vandewege, W., Wait Zaranek, A., & Wait Zaranek, S. (2024). *Arvados* [Go]. https://doi.org/10.5281/zenodo.6382942

Vivian, J., Rao, A. A., Nothaft, F. A., Ketchum, C., Armstrong, J., Novak, A., Pfeil, J., Narkizian, J., Deran, A. D., Musselman-Brown, A., Schmidt, H., Amstutz, P., Craft, B., Goldman, M., Rosenbloom, K., Cline, M., O'Connor, B., Hanna, M., Birger, C., … Paten, B. (2017). Toil enables reproducible, open source, big biomedical data analyses. *Nature Biotechnology, 35,* 314–316. https://doi.org/10.1038/nbt.3772

What is Airflow™?—Airflow Documentation. (n.d.). Retrieved February 23, 2024, from https://airflow.apache.org/docs/apache-airflow/stable/index.html

Wolstencroft, K., Haines, R., Fellows, D., Williams, A., Withers, D., Owen, S., Soiland-Reyes, S., Dunlop, I., Nenadic, A., Fisher, P., Bhagat, J., Belhajjame, K., Bacall, F., Hardisty, A., Nieva de la Hidalga, A., Balcazar Vargas, M. P., Sufi, S., & Goble, C. (2013). The Taverna workflow suite: Designing and executing workflows of Web Services on the desktop, web or in the cloud. *Nucleic Acids Research, 41*(W1), W557–W561. https://doi.org/10.1093/nar/gkt328

Zaharia, M., Chowdhury, M., Franklin, M. J., Shenker, S., & Stoica, I. (n.d.). *Spark: Cluster Computing with Working Sets.*

Chapter 4
Solution: Descriptive Dataflow Operators

This chapter proposes using descriptive dataflow operators to enhance workflow automation, especially in ETL pipelines beyond bioinformatics. Current descriptive languages inadequately address complex data transformations and data provenance, particularly at the granular level needed for healthcare regulations. Adopting a descriptive data modeling Domain-Specific Language (DSL) with a specialized syntax tailored for data processing tasks allows data transformations to be more efficiently compiled and documented, ensuring comprehensive data lineage and regulatory compliance.

After completing this chapter, readers should be able to:

1. Define the concept of descriptive dataflow operators
2. Explain the meaning of validation in the context of data processing pipelines

Adoption of Workflow DSLs Beyond Bioinformatics

While descriptive workflow languages have become the standard in domains like bioinformatics, dramatically increasing portability and reproducibility, their success has not yet translated to general data science or health informatics specifically. Many gaps still exist in addressing the processing needs of these broader fields.

First, the uptake of these languages has stalled in data preparation processes typical of ETL and ELT pipelines. One reason is that these languages rely on file-based processing architectures—often managing thousands of small files on a distributed file system. This paradigm contrasts sharply with ETL and, especially, ELT workflows, which primarily operate on database objects and diverse data sources. Furthermore, implementations of CWL, WDL and Nextflow offer advanced functionality when handling specific, well-defined file formats (such as FASTA/Q, BAM/CRAM

M. Bouzinier et al., *Research Data that Can Be Trusted*,
SpringerBriefs in Computer Science, https://doi.org/10.1007/978-3-032-21032-6_4

or VCF in bioinformatics); similar functionality is lacking outside that niche. Consequently, generalizing their input and output definitions to accommodate the heterogeneous data structures found in databases (such as scalar values, tables, or collections) is not straightforward.

We should also keep in mind that descriptive workflow languages work best when data operators (nodes of a DAG) are expected to come from a limited set of commonly used tools, as happens in bioinformatics. The fact that these tools are known and documented, with the knowledge of how to orchestrate them often built into the workflow orchestration frameworks, makes the operators less black boxes when a descriptive workflow language is used for a bioinformatics pipeline.

Conversely, ETL processes frequently encounter complex data transformations that are obscured by poorly readable programming languages such as Structured Query Language (SQL) or Perl. When performing traditional data transformations in fields beyond bioinformatics, such as population health research, the data often come from a wider range of sources and in diverse and incompatible formats. Required transformations are performed with tools unknown to the framework and commonly, custom R or Python scripts are written for a specific project. Other data transformations are optimally performed as part of ETL inside a Database Management System (DBMS) and expressed in a language native to the DBMS, such as Transact-SQL for Microsoft SQL Server, PL/pgSQL for PostgreSQL and others. These factors obscure the DAG nodes, making them true black boxes.

Workflow DSLs and Data Provenance

It is also important that existing workflow definition languages lack the expressiveness necessary for comprehensive data provenance tracking—a critical requirement in regulated environments like healthcare. The data lineage they can provide is at the level of datasets, while we often need a data lineage at the level of a column within a dataset (column-level lineage) and at an individual data element (cell-level lineage), referring to a cell as the intersection of a row and column in a data table.

Finally, modern regulatory frameworks demand not just automation but also detailed documentation of data transformations, quality controls and validation steps. This gap becomes particularly evident when dealing with healthcare data processing pipelines that must demonstrate compliance with multiple regulatory requirements.

Our Proposition: Dataflow Operators as the Next Level of Abstraction

To address these issues, we propose augmenting current methodologies by advancing to a higher abstraction level with the introduction of descriptive dataflow operators. This approach promises to improve readability, expressiveness and adaptability, better serving the nuanced requirements of ETL and general research workflows.

A significant advantage of this abstraction is the ability to map data lineage meticulously—from each input through every transformation to each eventual output—thereby constructing comprehensive column-level and cell-level lineage graphs.

Our proposal is based on the fact that each operator is a program written in a programming language. Most often, it is written in a procedural language, sometimes in a functional language. What if instead they were expressed in a descriptive programming language? While procedural languages outline each step like a recipe, descriptive ones specify the final result without detailing every cooking step, leaving it to implementations to decide on the most efficient step sequences in a given environment. We have already discussed that workflow definition languages have many features of a descriptive language. Another example of a descriptive language is SQL. As a descriptive language should do, it describes the desired outcome, but not the step-by-step process to achieve it. For instance, a simple SQL query describes the conditions that records must meet to be included in the result set. Various Query Planners translate an SQL document into executable code appropriate for a specific environment. Oracle Query Planner generates code different from the PostgreSQL Query Planner. For the same SQL query, the resulting code is even more different for hierarchical DBMSs like InterSystems IRIS or columnar DBMSs like Apache Druid (*Introduction to Apache Druid | Apache® Druid* n.d.). It is even more different for columnar databases like DuckDB (Raasveldt and Mühleisen 2019) that directly use a file system to store the data. If we could unambiguously describe the data transformations that occur in every dataflow operator, these could then be compiled into efficient executable code appropriate for a specific data platform, whether it be an SQL-compatible DBMS or the Hadoop Distributed File System (HDFS).

Based on these considerations, we see merits in adopting a descriptive language for dataflow operators—a data modeling DSL. We suggest that descriptive programming languages provide an ideal foundation for implementing sophisticated data provenance capabilities. By their nature, descriptive languages focus on declaring transformations and relationships rather than procedural steps, making them particularly well-suited for capturing detailed data lineage and validation requirements demanded by healthcare regulations.

One can argue that SQL is already a descriptive data transformation language. However, SQL is primarily designed to describe constraints rather than transformations and it is mainly used with relational data. Another downside of SQL is that it does not explicitly define inputs and outputs, thus making it difficult to use for constructing fine-grained data lineage. We believe we need a more human-readable and more expressive language to address modern data provenance requirements.

To validate this approach, we developed a descriptive DSL, demonstrating its practical application through analysis of Medicare claims data from the Centers for Medicare & Medicaid Services (CMS). Our implementation shows how descriptive programming enables both precise specification of data transformations and comprehensive documentation of data provenance.

The following sections present our technical framework that leverages descriptive programming to implement granular data provenance. We evaluate this approach using the Medicare claims analysis, demonstrating how it enables both efficient data processing and the detailed provenance documentation required in regulated healthcare environments. The regulatory implications are discussed in Part III.

Three Types of Validation

Validation is a heavily overloaded term. When discussing data transformations and a language that describes them, we should distinguish three types of validation:

- **Data quality validation** ensures that the raw data obtained from primary sources are consumable by processing algorithms. A common practice in data engineering is to simply discard records that are not consumable; however, more sophisticated approaches are also possible, e.g., attempting to correct invalid values. Examples of invalid values are numerics and dates out of range (e.g., a date of patient visit that has occurred 1000 years ago), invalid characters in numeric fields, or non-conformance to predefined patterns in fields (e.g. Social Security numbers).
- **Validation of algorithms** ensures that the processing of the data produces the results that correspond to the specifications. The simplest example is to validate that the average age for a set of three people with ages 2, 20 and 80 years is equal to 34.
- **Validation of constraints** ensures that data processing workflows are conformant with certain imposed requirements. For example, if a preprocessing pipeline is used to construct a training dataset for an AI model, we may require that the resulting dataset include representative population groups (e.g., both males and females and people of different ages). Alternatively, a constraint might stipulate that people under the age of 18 must be excluded from the training set for regulatory reasons. In theory, validation of constraints is possible even without actual data, by checking the logic of the workflow against the specified constraints.

A language describing data transformations must include **data quality validation** operators and we will discuss such operators in Chap. 5 Language Design section. **Validation of algorithms** can be performed using automated, detailed data lineage. A data lineage graph can also generate simple, explainable code to process a small set of raw values where the result is known a priori. We discuss it in the Fine-grained Data Lineage section of Chap. 5. **Validation of constraints** while being out of scope of this book can be included in a language in the form of annotations referring to invariants that must be preserved during transformations (Leavens and Cheon 2006; Mraihi et al. 2013).

References

Introduction to Apache Druid | Apache® Druid. (n.d.). Retrieved February 23, 2024, from https://druid.apache.org/docs/latest/design/

Leavens, G. T., & Cheon, Y. (2006). *Design by Contract with JML* (Nos. TR06-15). Iowa State University.

Mraihi, O., Louhichi, A., Jilani, L. L., Desharnais, J., & Mili, A. (2013). Invariant assertions, invariant relations, and invariant functions. *Science of Computer Programming, 78*(9), 1212–1239. https://doi.org/10.1016/j.scico.2012.05.006

Raasveldt, M., & Mühleisen, H. (2019). DuckDB: An Embeddable Analytical Database. *Proceedings of the 2019 International Conference on Management of Data*, 1981–1984. https://doi.org/10.1145/3299869.3320212

Chapter 5
Language Design

This chapter outlines the design of a domain-specific language (DSL) for healthcare data processing, which addresses technical efficiency and regulatory compliance. The DSL leverages a structured methodology similar to Medallion Architecture, transforming raw data into analytics-ready datasets while ensuring comprehensive data provenance. Key elements include dataset operators, field construction operators and validation operators to maintain data integrity. The language supports detailed cell-level and row-level lineage, providing transparency and compliance in healthcare data workflows.

After completing this chapter, readers should be able to:

1. Construct dataset operators for healthcare data processing
2. Implement basic validation rules in workflow automation
3. Design workflows that maintain comprehensive data lineage
4. Implement validation operators for maintaining data integrity
5. Design workflows that support cell-level and row-level lineage

High-Level Data Modeling DSL Architecture

The design of a domain-specific language for healthcare data processing must address both technical requirements for efficient data transformation and regulatory requirements for comprehensive provenance tracking. Modern healthcare regulations demand granular documentation of data lineage, validation steps and quality controls throughout the data lifecycle. This dual requirement—technical efficiency and detailed provenance—shapes our language design choices, particularly in how we specify data transformations and capture their relationships.

The Data Modeling DSL provides a structured methodology to transform heterogeneous raw data into clean, consistent datasets suitable for research and business analytics, while maintaining detailed records of all transformations for regulatory

M. Bouzinier et al., *Research Data that Can Be Trusted*,
SpringerBriefs in Computer Science, https://doi.org/10.1007/978-3-032-21032-6_5

compliance. Our methodology supports both the technical needs of data processing and the documentation requirements of regulated healthcare environments.

Although developed independently, our methodology mirrors aspects of Medallion Architecture (*What Is a Medallion Architecture?* 2022). We employ an iterative, multi-tiered data processing to facilitate data refinement through successive operations, transitioning from raw to advanced analytic-ready datasets. Each transformation is documented, enabling detailed provenance tracking from source data through all processing steps. Raw datasets undergo initial cleansing and augmentation to produce derivative datasets. These datasets form a chain, each iteration refining the data further, culminating in advanced datasets suitable for ML, AI, statistical analysis and business analytics.

Downstream datasets depend on upstream data; these dependencies can be efficiently visualized as a DAG, which guides execution order and enables concurrency via a workflow definition language. Our model pairs a workflow language, which specifies the DAG topology, with a data modeling language, which specifies what each node does. In this approach, nodes are dataset operators that, in turn, use field-construction operators to transform individual fields (for example, columns in relational tables). To design a data modelling DSL—that is a language syntax that allows us to define the semantics of these operators precisely—we first need to analyze the most common types of data transformations.

Transformations are functions, which have expected input types. In the iterative process of data preparation, transformations are chained and it is important to validate that the outputs of an upstream transformation are compatible with the expected input type of the downstream transformation. Further in this section, we will analyze the most common datatypes used in data cleansing and augmentation. Having classified the most common types of data transformations and the datatypes used by their processing functions, we can design an appropriate data modeling language.

Validation is essential for maintaining the accuracy and reliability of the final datasets from the data manipulation framework. This process, although it may sound tedious, ensures the integrity and provenance of datasets as they undergo successive transformations.

By systematically classifying data transformations and aligning them with validation practices, we lay the groundwork for a robust and efficient data modeling language.

Dataset Operator

A dataset operator, represented as a node in the dataflow DAG, takes a collection of datasets as input and produces another collection of datasets as output. A good practice is to presume that input datasets are immutable, i.e., operators do not modify any datasets but only produce new ones. This presumption ensures idempotency of every operator and potentially allows restarting the workflow from any point.

A dataset consists of records and each record contains data elements. We assume these elements conform to a defined schema and we refer to them as *fields*. For example, in a relational DBMS or a comma-separated values (CSV) file, a field corresponds to a column. In a document database such as MongoDB, a field can be more flexible and versatile.

In general, a dataset operator creates values for each field in the output records by taking values from fields in the input records and transforming them. An important assumption we make is that any new value depends only on input values, not on values computed by other field-construction operators in the same dataset operator.

There is one exception: it is possible to add new fields that are computed purely from other fields in the **same output record** and thus can be expressed as generated columns in SQL. For example, within the same logical dataset we might construct two new fields: **dob** (date of birth) and **age**. Construction of **dob** may require harmonization, normalization and cleansing, possibly involving aggregations such as building a master beneficiaries index. Once a clean **dob** is available, however, **age** is a simple deterministic function of that field. In PostgreSQL, **age** can be defined as a generated column such as:

```
age integer
  GENERATED ALWAYS AS (
    "YEAR" - EXTRACT(year FROM dob)
  ) STORED,
```

We will refer to the operation of creating a data element as a ‘***field construction operator***’.

Therefore, a dataset operator:

- operates on immutable datasets
- is a union of field construction operators
- combines field-construction operators that operate independently of one another and can be applied in any order.

The structure of a dataset operator consists of 3 elements:

- A list of inputs
- An immutable function or expression that calculates the new values
- A list of outputs.

For ‘***field construction operator***’, however, we expect a single output value. Single value, though, can be a collection, e.g., a PostgreSQL Array type. Exceptionally, the outputs of the unnesting operator and of transposing columns are values distributed over multiple rows.

Datatypes

As mentioned above, a description of an operator must include a list of its inputs. Each input element can be either a single value or a set. It is important to note, that a single value can also be a collection (e.g., a PostgreSQL Array type). A set is typically defined by a filter or a condition that selects certain records from an input dataset and extracts certain fields from the selected records. Operators that use sets as input are usually referred to as ***aggregations***.

Whether an input element is a single value (including collections) or a set, it has a certain type. It is important to know the type of input in order to optimize the execution of the operator. Every DBMS supports a variety of physical types, such as strings, integer or float values, dates, etc. However, for dataset operators, knowing physical types is insufficient to efficiently execute an operator. They could be optimized further by providing logical types. For example, a physical type of ***string*** (or, VARCHAR in SQL) can represent any of the following logical types:

- Id: a logical type that is assumed to be a relatively short string, unique in a certain scope. In a record it is either a unique identifier for this record or a reference to another record in the same or another dataset.
- Name: a logical type that is assumed to be a relatively short string referring to a human readable identifier (not necessarily unique) of a record. Names often appear in searches and filters and thus are usually being indexed. They are often used in ordering clauses when records retrieved by a query have to come in a specific order.
- Text: possibly a long string, consisting of tokens. There is no sense in indexing texts as whole strings, however, they are often indexed using special indices, for example by indexing tokens within the text.
- UUID or GUID: An id that is globally unique.
- URL or URI: a reference to a resource, complying to a certain template.
- Categorical value: a string that in this context can have only a few distinct values. Categorical fields are usually indexed and can be indexed using bitmap indices. They are often used in conditions for aggregations.

Next, we will review the types of field construction operators we have identified.

Types of Field Construction Operators

Data transformations can be categorized into two primary types: those that operate on a single value and those that manipulate multiple values by applying specific rules. This section will explore these categories, beginning with single-value transformations.

Here we introduce only as much of the transformation taxonomy as is needed to understand the language design and implementation in Chaps. 6, 7, 8 and 9. A more complete and formal classification, with additional examples, is provided in Part IV for readers interested in the technical details of DSL design or implementation.

Table 5.1 presents a summary of field construction operators while Part IV (Chap. 14) is dedicated to the detailed discussion.

Table 5.1 Field construction operators

Transformation type	Input dataset(s)	Input value	Output	Processing method	Reversible?
Isomorphic transformation	Single dataset	Single value	Single value	Arbitrary function or expression written in a procedural language, or as a valid SQL expression	Yes
Non-isomorphic transformation (including normalization)	Single dataset	Single value	Single value	Arbitrary function or expression written in a procedural language, or as a valid SQL expression	No, involves loss of information
Rollup	Single dataset	Single value	Single value	Mapping many-to-one function	No (loss of information)
Union transformation	Multiple datasets	Single value	Single value	Field alignment, type casting and copying	Yes
Approximation	Single dataset	Single value	Single or multiple value(s)	Arbitrary function	No (possible loss of information)
Simple aggregation	Single dataset	Multiple values	Single value	Built-in aggregation function	No
Custom aggregation	Single dataset	Multiple values	Single value	User provided aggregation function	No
Flattening arrays	Single dataset	Multiple values	Single value	Built-in aggregation function	Yes
Unnesting of arrays	Single dataset	Single value	Multiple values	Unnest function	Yes
Collapsing multiple columns into arrays	Single dataset	Multiple values (horizontal)	Single value (array)	Combine into an array	Yes
Transposing columns to rows	Single dataset	Multiple values (horizontal)	Multiple values (vertical)	Combine into an array and unnest	Yes

Disambiguation Rules for Aggregations

Aggregations often require disambiguation rules, particularly when the expected output is a single value but the aggregation results in a set of multiple, potentially conflicting values. Such scenarios necessitate specific disambiguation rules, which should be expressible within the data transformation DSL.

Example:

For each Medicare beneficiary, for certain data points like date of birth (DOB), sex, race, ethnicity and date of death (DOD) we expect a single value per field. However, discrepancies often arise in enrollment records, necessitating a strategy for handling such ambiguities. When it happens, the rule raises the ambiguity flag that can be recorded along with the data. Here are some disambiguation rules for managing these variances:

- **DOB**: Select the earliest DOB from the enrollment records for the primary value. Additionally, track the latest DOB as a secondary value in a separate column, setting it to NULL when DOB is unambiguous.

  From the data analyzed between 1999 and 2018, approximately 0.27% of beneficiaries exhibited ambiguous DOBs. Typically, excluding these beneficiaries from datasets is advisable unless necessary to include them—where recording the latest DOB aids in age verification.

  Most discrepancies arise from minor errors (e.g., within 10 days) or errors in the month or year, likely due to paperwork mistakes. Mismatches not aligning with these patterns may indicate the mixing of records from distinct beneficiaries.
- **DOD**: The rule is similar to DOB disambiguation but excludes NULLs from aggregations, as DOD is naturally NULL for records dated prior to a beneficiary's death. The actual rule is: select the latest recorded DOD and document the earliest DOD separately.
- **Race, ethnicity and sex**: use string aggregation for distinct values. However, adoption of more refined rules may be necessary based on user feedback. For instance, if a value is consistent across all but one enrollment year, it might be practical to default to the prevailing value, treating anomalies as artefacts. DSL should allow for such configurations, including setting thresholds on allowable record variances.

Data Validation Operators

Preventing Systematic Errors and Biases

The primary objective of a data warehouse, especially one supporting ML and AI models, is to provide a clean and consistent dataset that meets regulatory standards. Raw data sourced from various origins often contains gaps, inconsistencies and discrepancies that need to be addressed through data cleansing. It is crucial to ensure that the cleansing process does not introduce systematic errors, thereby preserving the integrity and avoiding bias of the research conclusions or model predictions. To avert such issues and maintain regulatory compliance, careful validation approaches are necessary, with a focus on documenting decisions to exclude certain records that fail to meet validation criteria from the final dataset.

Key Validation Checks

1. **Primary Key Integrity**: Ensure that each record contains non-null data for all attributes required to form a valid primary key.
2. **Consistency Across Records**: Verify that records remain consistent with one another within the data warehouse. For instance, in processing a Medicaid claim record for an inpatient admission, ensure the beneficiary was enrolled in Medicaid at the time of admission. This step involves validating foreign keys and cross-references.
3. **Elimination of Duplicates**: Check that records are unique and not inadvertently duplicated or counted multiple times.

Handling Validation Failures

When a record fails validation checks, specific actions must be taken. Options include ignoring such records or logging them in a special journal for quality control (QC) reporting.

The data manipulation Domain-Specific Language (DSL) should support defining these actions, including specifying the target datastore for records that fail validation if they are to be retained for further review or analysis.

Fine-Grained Data Lineage

Data Lineage and Algorithmic Validation

Robust data lineage provides transparency and validation for ethical and regulatory conformant research outcomes. Fine-grained lineage serves two crucial purposes: enhancing explainability by meticulously tracing every adjustment and transformation applied to compute each data point and bolstering trust in the data by generating transparent and understandable procedures that facilitate manual validation of selected data points. This validation can be applied either to random selection or to specific outliers, thereby identifying potential bugs and systematic errors in processing workflows.

Achieving a granular level of data lineage in complex datasets requires both row-level and column-level tracking. Conventional tools often only support dataset-level lineage, but regulatory compliance and ethical considerations in healthcare demand traceability down to individual cell values.

Achieving Cell-Level Lineage

For cell-level provenance, a construction of both row-level and column-level lineage is necessary. This is made possible through the integration of dataflow programming concepts into the data modeling DSL. The column-level data lineage can be derived from analyzing the field construction operators, which articulate how each field in a dataset is derived from fields in upstream datasets. Visual representation of this process can be structured as a DAG of operators, providing a clear overview of how each data point is processed and documented for compliance purposes.

Directives for Row-Based Lineage

Implementing the DSL requires specific directives to support row-level lineage. Two such directives have been introduced to ensure seamless tracking of data through every transformation stage, preserving the integrity and origin of each dataset element:

- **FILE Directive** instructs a data loader to add a field recording the original file URI from which the data has been ingested.
- **RECORD Directive** provides a unique reference for each record within the file.

Unified Approach for Holistic Lineage

Combining tools for the cell-level lineage with the directives for the row-based one forms a foundation for a comprehensive lineage strategy, ensuring that datasets remain fully auditable throughout their lifecycle. Further tools can potentially trace every value in the final dataset back to the original raw data values. When the final dataset is used for training AI models, combining these provenance tools with explainability techniques, such as Shapley (SHapley Additive exPlanations) Values (Lundberg and Lee 2017), can help ensure that the resulting models adhere to ethical principles and regulations.

References

Lundberg, S. M., & Lee, S.-I. (2017). A Unified Approach to Interpreting Model Predictions. *Advances in Neural Information Processing Systems, 30*. https://papers.nips.cc/paper_files/paper/2017/hash/8a20a8621978632d76c43dfd28b67767-Abstract.html

What is a Medallion Architecture? (2022, March 9). Databricks. https://www.databricks.com/glossary/medallion-architecture

Part II
How to Implement It

Chapter 6
Proof of Concept Implementation

The Dorieh Data Platform is Apache-licensed open-source software that exemplifies implementing a DSL-based approach for healthcare data processing, aligning with previously discussed concepts. Developed by Harvard, it incorporates Medallion Architecture principles to manage multi-level data lineage and maintain data confidentiality. The platform supports reproducible workflows using CWL for workflow topologies and a YAML-based DSL for precise data transformations. It integrates validation, journaling and automated documentation tools to enhance data quality, regulatory compliance and transparency.

After completing this chapter, readers should be able to:

1. Describe the architectural choices involved in building a modern data platform for healthcare data provenance.
2. Explain the role of Medallion Architecture principles in supporting reproducible, auditable data workflows.
3. Summarize the purpose and composition of a data domain definition file in the Dorieh data platform.
4. Construct and interpret dataset validation and journaling mechanisms within Dorieh to ensure data integrity and quality control.
5. Apply the Data Dictionary Generation tool to automatically produce comprehensive, human- and machine-readable documentation and visualize data lineage at both the table and column levels.
6. Evaluate the advantages and limitations of the Dorieh data platform approach to lineage and provenance, comparing it to other available solutions.

M. Bouzinier et al., *Research Data that Can Be Trusted*,
SpringerBriefs in Computer Science, https://doi.org/10.1007/978-3-032-21032-6_6

Choice of Technology: Backend, Workflow Engine and Language Syntax

A modern data platform for health data provenance must address both efficient data processing and rigorous auditability. This requires a foundation built on four pillars: (1) robust storage, (2) a scalable backend to execute field construction operators, (3) a workflow engine to orchestrate the execution of these operators and (4) a clear, expressive data modeling language to specify the transformations. Each of these components directly supports or constrains the platform's ability to deliver transparent, repeatable and auditable data pipelines.

Obviously, common data engineering tasks expressed as field construction operators can theoretically be accomplished using a wide array of programming languages and tools: procedural languages (C/C++, Python, Scala), data-centric libraries such as Pandas ("Pandas Documentation—Pandas 2.3.3 Documentation," n.d.), specialized programming languages such as R ("R: The R Project for Statistical Computing," n.d.) or even descriptive query languages like SQL. However, most widely adopted data manipulation tools (e.g., Pandas, R data frames) operate primarily in-memory, which limits their scalability for large datasets and can compromise reproducibility or provenance by making it difficult to track or audit data transformations at scale. Many advanced data transformations require joins including self-joins. Joins are Cartesian products of the datasets and thus exponentially increase memory requirements. For instance, a self-join on a dataset with one million records theoretically yields a billion-row intermediate table; a billion-row dataset could not be processed feasibly in memory on any realistic hardware. Such operations underscore the need for backends that efficiently handle data on disk or in distributed storage.

To overcome these technical barriers, two dominant architectures are used in modern data platforms:

Traditional Database Management Systems (DBMS), which leverage on-disk storage and optimize for high-throughput, transactional operations (increasingly using SSDs for speed) and

Resilient Distributed Datasets (RDDs) (Zaharia et al. 2012), as popularized by Apache Spark, which support parallel, fault-tolerant processing across multiple nodes.

Data platforms vary: some leverage robust third-party backends (e.g., Databricks uses Spark, SSIS uses SQL Server, Informatica and Talend can connect to a third-party backend like an RDBMS and/or Spark), while others—like Snowflake—build and maintain proprietary engines to deliver both storage and compute.

The majority of general-purpose data platforms as well as more specialized data platforms outside bioinformatics use their own proprietary workflow orchestration engines. Some platforms allow integration with data modeling tools such as dbt from dbt Labs (dbt Labs n.d.).

For the data modeling layer, YAML and JSON are leading choices due to their human- and machine-readability and ease of integration with workflow engines.

In Dorieh's initial, proof-of-concept implementation, PostgreSQL serves as the storage backend, and workflows are managed and orchestrated through the Common Workflow Language (CWL) engine. To maintain consistency with CWL, field construction operators are defined using a YAML/JSON-based domain-specific language (DSL). This arrangement provides a sufficient level of scalability while being open-source and enables the reproducibility, auditability and fine-grained lineage required for secondary health data uses. Future work includes integrating Apache Spark as an alternative backend, supporting a Groovy-based DSL for richer expressivity and enabling Nextflow for advanced workflow orchestration.

Dorieh Data Platform

The Dorieh Data Platform, developed by Harvard University Research Computing in collaboration with the National Studies for Air Pollution and Health (NSAPH), functions as a specialized data warehouse designed primarily as a feature store for the development of statistical models in population and environmental health research. Its core aim is to support reproducible research while safeguarding confidential data, emphasizing the importance of shareable workflows.

Mirroring Medallion Architecture (Databricks 2022), Dorieh ensures comprehensive data lineage and efficient data ingestion, with support for transformations fully managed within a DBMS. This architecture promotes the preservation of data lineage at table, row and column levels. Dorieh adopts an "as-is" ingestion policy, facilitated by its Introspection and Ingestion Module and discourages transformations during ingestion.

Dorieh supports multiple programming languages, such as Python, R and Java, for creating analytical tools. It includes a testing framework that verifies workflows through table fingerprinting, thereby ensuring data integrity. Documentation processes are streamlined through automated generation of Markdown and DOT files (Graphviz n.d.) for workflow documentation and data lineage graphs, ensuring consistency between code and documentation.

An embedded Geographic Information System (GIS) library provides capabilities for handling geographic data. The platform supports deployment via PyPi or Docker containers. It offers data import from various popular formats, such as CSV, fixed-width format (FWF), SAS File Transfer Summaries (FTS), SAS7BDAT, FST and JSONlines and allows data export to formats like FTS, CSV, Parquet and HDF5.

Dorieh employs the CWL for defining dataset operation topologies in data processing workflows. It also implements an initial version of a YAML-based data modeling DSL, which describes individual transformations. The data model definitions in YAML are partially compiled into SQL and Data Definition Language (DDL) and are partially interpreted by the Data Loader module at runtime to maintain consistency during data ingestion.

While the workflow definition language captures operational topology and provides a dataset-level data lineage graph, the data domain definition files offer column-level data lineage graphs. The design and implementation of the DSL was an iterative process that occurred in parallel development phases. As a result, not every field construction operator described previously has a dedicated syntax construct in the DSL. However, all field construction operators are expressible within the DSL, except for union transformations, which require additional DSL extensions as described below.

Dorieh Data Modeling DSL: Structure of a Domain Definition File

The Dorieh data modeling DSL is designed to precisely define the structure and transformation processes within a data warehouse, tailored for specific knowledge domains. Central to this specification is the concept of a domain, which encompasses datasets represented as tables. These tables are detailed within the tables directive of the domain definition.

Key Directives

Domain Directive. The foundational element, *domain*, dictates the organizational structure and transformation processes of datasets. Domains can specify default parameters, including SQL schema names and indexing policies.

Tables Directive. This directive outlines the construction of datasets and is located within the domain element. Tables can be categorized into root and child tables. Root tables serve as independent datasets, while child tables are linked via foreign keys, forming a tree-like hierarchy. Collectively, the domain definition creates a forest-like setup of interconnected tables. Each dataset within the tables directive specifies its type (e.g., true tables, views, or materialized views in an RDBMS) and includes a definition of the procedure for building the dataset.

Columns Directive. Each table component includes a columns directive, defining individual fields through field construction operators. These operators describe the logic for transforming input data fields into the desired output format.

Dorieh Domains and Databricks Delta Live Tables

A forest-like setup of interconnected tables is conceptually similar to the Databricks Delta Live Tables (DLT). The main difference is that while a DLT is always a materialized view, Dorieh allows intermediate datasets to be of any type. They can be true tables to support foreign keys or they can be lightweight views to avoid spending resources on actual computation.

Another important difference is that for DLT every dataset operator is either an SQL statement or a Python function. Dorieh uses a declarative approach to define dataset operators, making complex transformations easier to read and understand by humans and clearly defined for tools to automatically produce data dictionaries and data column-level lineage graphs.

Validation and Journaling

In the Dorieh Data Platform, validation and journaling are important components ensuring the integrity and quality of datasets within the data warehouse. These processes help in identifying and addressing gaps, inconsistencies, errors and anomalies in data, thereby preserving the reliability of research outcomes.

Validation

Purpose: Validation ensures that each record in a newly constructed dataset meets predefined criteria and standards. It checks for data correctness, consistency and completeness, safeguarding against the introduction of errors during data processing.

Default Behavior: By default, if any record fails validation checks, the system generates an error and the transaction for dataset creation is rolled back. This rollback mechanism prevents the inclusion of invalid data in the final dataset.

Customization: The DSL provides the flexibility to override default validation behavior on a per-dataset basis through the *invalid.records* directive. This allows for custom validation rules tailored to specific datasets or research needs.

Journaling

Policy Options: The platform offers two possible policies for handling records that fail validation: ignoring such records or journaling them in a separate table.

Journaling Process: If the journaling policy is selected, all records that fail validation are stored in a special audit table. Each entry is documented with annotations describing the specific reasons for validation failure and pointers to the related data.

Use Case: Journaling provides a valuable audit trail, allowing researchers to review and analyze why certain records did not meet validation criteria. This feature facilitates transparency in data handling and supports quality control efforts.

By integrating validation and journaling, the Dorieh Data Platform ensures that users can maintain high-quality datasets while also documenting and understanding data discrepancies. This dual approach balances strict data integrity with practical insights into data quality issues.

The Data Dictionary Generation Tool

Purpose

The Data Dictionary Generation Tool is an essential component of the Dorieh Data Platform, designed to streamline the documentation of data elements and facilitate clear insight into data lineage within the platform. By extracting and leveraging original documentation from the ingested data sources the tool automatically generates comprehensive documentation, thereby increasing transparency and usability for researchers and data analysts.

Key Features

Automated Documentation: The tool extracts documentation accompanying raw data sources and generates detailed documentation for all data elements, including tables and columns within the data model. This process minimizes manual work and reduces the risk of documentation errors.

Data Lineage Diagrams: It produces data lineage diagrams at both the table and column levels, illustrating the flow and transformation of data through the system. These diagrams are available in various image formats, such as PNG, GIF, SVG and JPEG, to suit different presentation needs.

Table-level Lineage: A main table-level diagram presents the sequence of data processing steps and the dependencies between tables. When generated in SVG format, these diagrams allow for interactive exploration, with clickable elements linking directly to detailed table descriptions.

Column-level Lineage: Each column within a table is linked to a file that provides a detailed description of the column and its lineage. These descriptions document the derivation of each column from upstream data, facilitating in-depth understanding of data transformations.

Centralized Index: An alphabetical index lists all columns across all tables, showing every instance of each column throughout the database.

Conversion to HTML: The tool initially generates documentation in Markdown format, which can be converted to HTML for easy sharing and accessibility.

It supports two modes: standalone mode using Pandoc and a Sphinx mode for integration into Sphinx-generated documentation.

By automating the creation of a detailed data dictionary, the Data Dictionary Generation Tool enhances the coherence and accessibility of documentation within the Dorieh platform.

Detailed Domain Definition File Syntax

For a comprehensive understanding of the Domain Definition File Syntax used by the Dorieh data modeling DSL, we provide extensive supplementary documents. These documents include:

Detailed syntax description: Appendix A details the foundational syntax structure, covering basic constructs and their applications.

Extensions: Appendix B explores advanced syntax extensions, necessary for more complex transformations such as union transformations.

These guides are essential for users who wish to leverage the full potential of the Dorieh platform by enabling precise domain and dataset definitions. The documents provide illustrative examples and detailed guidelines to facilitate understanding.

Dorieh in Context: Comparing Data Lineage and Provenance Solutions

The Dorieh Data Platform demonstrates a modern, open-source approach to data lineage and provenance, integrating lessons learned from both commercial and academic data platforms while introducing several novel features.

Key Distinguishing Features of Dorieh

- **Fine-grained Data Lineage**: Unlike many platforms that offer lineage tracking only at the dataset or table level, Dorieh supports both column-level lineage graphs out of the box and is designed to enable cell-level lineage—an essential feature for regulatory compliance and granular AI/ML auditability.
- **Declarative DSL for Data Modeling**: Dorieh's YAML/JSON-based domain-specific language lets users specify data transformations in a human- and machine-readable way, facilitating transparent, repeatable workflows. This contrasts with workflow engines or SQL-centric tools that treat complex transformations as "black boxes."

- **Integrated Validation and Journaling**: Built-in support for validation checks and journaling of invalid records creates clear audit trails and supports robust quality control—features sometimes lacking or cumbersome in other solutions.
- **Automated Documentation**: The Data Dictionary Generation tool provides interactive, comprehensive documentation with lineage diagrams, supporting transparency and reducing the manual workload traditionally associated with regulatory compliance and reproducibility.
- **Medallion Architecture Principles**: Dorieh leverages an iterative, multi-tiered approach, mirroring established best practices in modern analytics platforms (such as Databricks Delta Live Tables), while allowing greater flexibility in the choice between views, tables and materialized views for intermediate datasets.

Dorieh and Other Solutions

- **Commercial Data Platforms (e.g., Databricks, Snowflake, Talend)**: These often provide integration with enterprise data warehouses and support scalable orchestration, but may obscure the details of data transformations or lineage, offer limited cell/column-level tracing and lock features behind proprietary code or licensing.
- **Bioinformatics Workflow Frameworks (e.g., CWL, Nextflow, Snakemake)**: While strong in automation and portable workflow definition, such tools often lack detailed provenance below the dataset level and are tied to file-based, batch-oriented processing models.
- **Custom or Ad Hoc Solutions**: Many research groups rely on pipelines combining scripts, notebooks and database queries, which can make lineage discovery and documentation labor-intensive and error-prone.

Current Limitations and Future Directions

Dorieh's DSL is evolving—some complex operations (e.g., union transformations) require additional syntax extensions and support for new backends and workflow orchestrators (like Spark and Nextflow) is under development. The ultimate goal is seamless, scalable cell-level provenance in any computing environment.

When to Consider Dorieh

Dorieh is an especially strong fit when regulatory compliance, reproducibility and transparency in health data workflows are paramount; when your team values automated, fine-grained documentation and lineage; or when you need an extensible, open-source platform that can adapt to evolving standards in healthcare AI.

References

Control plane for data collaboration at scale. (n.d.). Dbt Labs. Retrieved October 12, 2025, from https://www.getdbt.com/resources/whitepaper-the-control-plane-for-data-collaboration-at-scale

DOT Language. (n.d.). Graphviz. Retrieved October 13, 2024, from https://graphviz.org/doc/info/lang.html

pandas documentation—Pandas 2.3.3 documentation. (n.d.). Retrieved October 12, 2025, from https://pandas.pydata.org/docs/index.html

R: The R Project for Statistical Computing. (n.d.). Retrieved October 12, 2025, from https://www.r-project.org/

What is a Medallion Architecture? (2022, March 9). Databricks. https://www.databricks.com/glossary/medallion-architecture

Zaharia, M., Chowdhury, M., Das, T., Dave, A., Ma, J., McCauley, M., Franklin, M. J., Shenker, S., & Stoica, I. (2012). Resilient distributed datasets: A fault-tolerant abstraction for in-memory cluster computing. *Proceedings of the 9th USENIX Conference on Networked Systems Design and Implementation*, 2.

Chapter 7
Sample Application: Building ML-Ready Datasets

This chapter connects the architectural principles from Chap. 6 to a concrete, end-to-end example. We walk through the design of a small but realistic pipeline and show how Dorieh implements it using descriptive workflows and a data-modeling DSL.

To make the example easily reproducible by readers, we use **open gridded climate data aggregated over ZIP code areas** rather than restricted health data. In Chap. 8 we then apply the same design ideas to a real healthcare setting: Medicare claims.

A complete, step-by-step implementation of the climate pipeline—including full CWL and YAML files, commands and troubleshooting notes—is available as an online tutorial in the Dorieh GitHub repository. In this chapter we focus on the design and how it exemplifies the patterns introduced earlier.

After completing this chapter, readers will be able to:

1. Relate the abstract design principles from Chap. 6 to a concrete pipeline.
2. Describe how a descriptive workflow language and a data-modeling DSL work together in practice.
3. Explain how Bronze, Silver and Gold Layers support ML-ready dataset construction.
4. Understand, at a high level, how validation, journaling and documentation tools are wired into a workflow.
5. Use the online tutorial as a template for their own pipelines.

Designing a Pipeline

In the real world, many data workflows begin ad hoc and evolve reactively as requirements become clearer and more specific. This creates a feedback loop driving workflow evolution. When feasible, however, proactively designing a data pipeline produces workflows that are much easier to maintain, audit and scale—especially in regulated settings or for ML applications.

M. Bouzinier et al., *Research Data that Can Be Trusted*,
SpringerBriefs in Computer Science, https://doi.org/10.1007/978-3-032-21032-6_7

Even when requirements are not available upfront and proactive design is therefore not realistic, understanding the design process still helps you build an incremental ad hoc workflow in a cleaner, more structured way.

Once a pipeline is mature enough, it is not too late to apply design principles at a "cleanup" stage and refactor the pipeline to be more robust. In regulated domains, this kind of refactoring is ultimately unavoidable.

Designing a robust data workflow—and building implementations that follow that design—is an important prerequisite for reproducible research, data governance and ML-ready datasets. We therefore adopt a simple five-step design process for a Dorieh-based pipeline. These steps consider the nature of the data sources, required transformations, quality control and output requirements.

Step 1. Identify Data Sources and Producers

Begin by inventorying all input datasets and their origins. Data may come from:

- Heterogeneous sources: government agencies, commercial vendors, climate repositories, etc.
- Varied delivery mechanisms:
  - File downloads (CSV, FST, Parquet, HDF5, etc.)
  - Database or data warehouse connections (SQL-based)
  - Web APIs (e.g., REST endpoints)
- File access protocols: local, S3, HTTP/HTTPs, etc.

Each data producer may have its own update schedule, documentation standards and pre-processing conventions. Understanding these is essential to harmonize inputs and document provenance.

> *Dorieh Implementation Note: Dorieh currently offers built-in support for numerous common file formats and has basic connectors for several external databases and select APIs (e.g., climate, census). Supported file formats include, but are not limited to: CSV, FST, JSON, SAS7BDAT, FWF, Parquet, HDF5 including NetCDF. Supported APIs include: climate data from Climatology Lab, AirNow, limited support for Census, SQL connectors.*
>
> *For data types or APIs that are not natively supported, third-party components are easily integrated, especially when wrapped via CWL. CWL natively supports multiple file access protocols like S3 and HTTP/HTTPS.*

Step 2. Specify Data Consumers and Target Outputs

Next, clarify **who** will use the data and in **what form**:

- Who are the consumers? Data scientists, researchers, policy analysts, clinicians?

- What tools will consumers use to achieve their goals (BI, Notebooks, Dashboards, APIs)?
- What format(s) do these downstream tools require?
  - Database tables (in RDBMS, Spark warehouses, Iceberg),
  - Files (CSV/Parquet, HDF5)
  - REST endpoints
- What are the expectations for:
  - Data cleanliness and normalization
  - Documentation and traceability
  - Compliance reports or data dictionaries

By understanding consumer needs, you can tailor outputs to balance flexibility and efficiency.

Step 3. Map the Logical Dataflow

Design the logical steps needed to transform raw data into ML-ready, analytics-grade form. For each dataset:

- Define essential transformations:
  - **Normalization**: standardizing formats and code systems (e.g., state codes, date formats).
  - **Harmonization**: reconciling column names/types, resolving coding discrepancies across years or producers.
  - **Cleansing**: identifying and handling missing, implausible, or inconsistent values (e.g., negative ages, impossible dates).
- Establish quality control (QC) checkpoints to:
  - Detect outliers, duplicates and anomalies
  - Log data losses or errors for auditing (important for regulatory compliance)
- Plan for iterative, multi-layer transformation in accordance with medallion architecture:
  - **Bronze**: Raw, as-ingested data (minimal to no transformation)
  - **Silver**: Cleaned, harmonized and enriched data
  - **Gold**: Aggregated, analytic-ready datasets, possibly containing derived features

At each stage, explicitly think about **reproducibility** (can this step be repeated elsewhere?), **transparency** (can we explain it?) and **auditability** (can we show what happened?).

Step 4. Lay Out Workflow Topology

Using a workflow definition language (e.g., CWL or Nextflow):

- Define tasks and their dependencies: what runs before what and what data flows between them.
- Identify where parallelization (scatter, batching) is appropriate.
- Decide if data or compute needs are anticipated to grow, requiring scalability of the workflow to be incorporated into design. If yes, identify where parallelization (scatter, batching) is appropriate and how you will scale the workflow.
- Integrate validation, journaling and lineage-tracking mechanisms into each stage.

Remember that the workflow language describes the DAG topology—the nodes and edges—while the data-modeling DSL describes what each node does to the data.

Step 5. Plan Documentation and Provenance

Finally, ensure that each pipeline element supports:

- Automated schema and transformation documentation (via Dorieh's data-modeling DSL and dictionary tools)
- Generation of data lineage diagrams at the dataset and column levels
- Logging of all data quality actions and decisions—for auditing and reproducibility.

Summary of Design Decisions

The summary of the design process is reflected in Table 7.1.

Use Case: Aggregate Gridded Climate Data Over ZIP Code Areas

To see this design process in action, we use a climate-data example that is fully reproducible with open data. The eventual workflow will involve multiple sources, geospatial aggregation, transformations and ML-ready outputs.

The current Dorieh version leverages Common Workflow Language (CWL) to orchestrate processing tasks. The steps below demonstrate constructing a sample workflow to aggregate gridded climate data over ZIP code areas in the contiguous United States (lower 48 states), culminating in a multi-layer ("medallion") data model in PostgreSQL.

Table 7.1 Workflow design decisions

Phase	Main questions	Dorieh features involved
Source intake	Where does data originate? In what format? What's the update cycle?	Multi-format support, CWL inputs
QC/ETL	How to normalize, harmonize and cleanse? What's the error policy?	Validation operators, journaling
Output	Where and in what form is data consumed? What schemas are required?	Domain definition (YAMLDSL), CWL outputs
Workflow	What is the DAG topology and parallelism strategy?	CWL, Dorieh task wrappers
Documentation	How will provenance and data lineage be captured?	Workflow documentation utilities, data dictionary tool, automated lineage diagrams

Use Case Overview

- **Data producer**: Google Earth Engine
- **Input Sources**:
  - **Gridded temperature** from the Northwest Knowledge Network (NKN), University of Idaho (*IIDS NKN* n.d.). The temperature units are Kelvin.
  - ***Shape files*** *for geographic boundaries (ZIP Code Tabulation Areas, counties), obtained from U.S. Census sources. Note, this source is not included in the original requirements but is added later when we design the Essential Transformations step and realize that it is required for aggregation over geographic boundaries.*
- **Data consumer**: A researcher interested in climate characteristics of U.S. states and cities, possibly to build ML models relating climate to health or environmental outcomes.
- **Outputs**:
  - A CSV file where each record contains a date, a ZIP code (ZCTA) and an aggregated climate variable (e.g., daily maximum temperature).
  - A PostgreSQL database implementing a Bronze/Silver/Gold model, enabling efficient querying, visualization and ML feature extraction.

Essential Transformations

Working from the design steps:

1. **Aggregation over geographic boundaries**

- The raw NKN data are on a climate grid. We must aggregate grid cells into ZIP code or county polygons.
- This is easier to perform outside the DBMS, on files or in a geospatial engine; Dorieh includes a CWL-wrapped tool that does precisely this, using shape files.

2. **Unit conversion**
    - Convert temperatures from Kelvins to Celsius and Fahrenheit.
    - These are simple isomorphic transformations defined as field construction operators in the DSL.
3. **Geospatial enrichment**
    - Annotate each ZIP code with state abbreviations and (where applicable) city names, using built-in lookup functions (e.g., zip_to_state, zip_to_city).
4. **State-level aggregation**
    - Aggregate ZIP-level readings into state-level summaries per date: mean temperature and temperature span (max–min) across ZIPs.

Workflow Topology

- Data acquisition
- Preparation for ingestion
- Ingestion into the database
- Performing Silver Layer transformations
- Building Gold Layer.

Bronze, Silver and Gold in This Example

Applied to the climate use case:

- **Bronze Layer**
    - Contains one table, bronze_temperature.
    - Each record represents a (date, ZCTA) pair with a raw temperature in Kelvin (tmmx).
    - This layer is produced by the CWL workflow's aggregation step and ingested into PostgreSQL using the Dorieh data loader.
    - The table's schema is defined declaratively in YAML, including primary keys and basic field metadata.
- **Silver Layer**

  - Contains an enriched view silver_temperature built from the Bronze table.
  - Adds:

    Temperature in Celsius and Fahrenheit (temperature_in_C, temperature_in_F).

    State abbreviation (us_state) and city (city) derived from the ZCTA and date via lookup functions.
  - This is defined in the data-modeling DSL as a view with field construction operators expressing these transformations.

- **Gold Layer**
  - Contains a materialized view gold_temperature_by_state.
  - Groups by (us_state, date) and computes:

    Mean temperature in Celsius and Fahrenheit.

    Temperature span (t_span) as MAX(tmmx) – MIN(tmmx) across ZIPs within the state.
  - This layer is ML- and analytics-ready: you can plug it into modeling pipelines, dashboards, or export it as files.

Implementing the Pipeline

Building CWL Pipelines

Dorieh includes a collection of built-in CWL tools that we will be leveraging in our examples.

It is also possible to wrap your own Python script (or anything else that can be run in a command line) as a CWL tool. There are tools like argparse2tool (Helena 2015/2025) that masquerade as argparse and attempt to find and import the real argparse. It then stores a reference to the code module for the system argparse and presents the user with all of the functions that stdlib's argparse provides. Every function call is passed through the system argparse. However, argparse2tool captures the details of those calls and when CWL is requested, it builds up the tool definition and prints it out to standard output.

A detailed Tutorial for building the data processing workflows is provided in Dorieh Online Documentation: https://foromeplatform.github.io/dorieh/tutorial/climate/building-climate-pipeline.html

In this section we will outline the six steps described in the tutorial.

Step 1. Initializing a Minimal CWL Workflow Skeleton

The goal of this step is to sketch out the overall pipeline in CWL without worrying yet about the exact parameters or data wiring. We can think of it as drawing a high-level flowchart: boxes (steps) exist, but the arrows (data connections) and concrete inputs/outputs are still missing. As a result, the workflow is not runnable yet, but it gives you a clear outline of the process.

The sequence of operations the pipeline will follow:

- First, get raw gridded climate data.
- Then, aggregate over ZCTA areas.

We will leverage the fact that Dorieh provides a library of prebuilt CWL tool definitions, streamlining common steps such as downloading remote files, fetching census geographies and running aggregations.

At this point, the workflow is not yet runnable; it simply outlines the main stages of the process (download, aggregate) as nodes in a future DAG.

Step 2. Iteratively Defining Steps and Parameters

In the second step we turn the skeleton into a runnable CWL workflow by formalizing each step's interface. For every tool, we identify required inputs (e.g., year, climate band, geography), declare outputs (data files, logs, error logs) and then wire them together in the workflow.

We start by examining documentation of each of the underlying tools, subsequently applying Dorieh's cwl_collect_outputs utility to generate consistent `out` and `outputs` sections from tool CWL definitions..

For example, transforming the download step from an abstract box into a well-specified operation that:

- Receives parameters that fully determine what data to fetch.
- Emits specific named files that other steps can consume.

We note that it needs:

- (Optionally) proxy settings.
- A year (e.g., 2019) that determines which time period to download.
- A climate variable (band), such as daily maximum temperature.

To handle these requirements we add "year" and "band" as workflow inputs (so the user can choose them when running the workflow) and connect those workflow inputs to the download step's inputs.

It is important to note that when inspecting the aggregation tool, we see that it also needs the shapes (ZCTA polygons), not just the climate grid. It prompts us to add another step that uses a Dorieh shapes-download tool (get_shapes) to fetch ZCTA shapefiles for the right year.

Practically, at this step, we construct a **dataflow**:

- The download step produces the raw climate data.
- The get_shapes step produces the spatial boundaries.

- The aggregate step consumes both and produces a table of daily values per ZCTA.

By defining inputs/outputs and wiring, we instruct CWL on the execution order and file passing: which file from which step is given to which input of another step. At this point the workflow can be run for a full year of data. Notably, there is now no hidden behavior: every dependency and file flow is explicit in the CWL.

Step 3. Testing with Minimal Data Slices

The workflow constructed in step 2 is a runnable workflow for a full year of data. However, full-year runs can be very slow, so the next step introduces a "toy" (single-day) mode. At the next step we make development and debugging faster by allowing the pipeline to run on a very small dataset, typically for just one day instead of an entire year.

We need to add a date for which to perform the aggregation to the workflow inputs. This makes the explicit year parameter redundant because the date includes the year. The problem is though that the tools we are using do require a year to download the data correctly. Hence, we need to add a simple data-transformation node, that does not talk to any external systems but just transforms one input (a text date) into another (a year number). Conceptually, we now have layers of parameters:

- Human-friendly input (date), which is easier to reason about during development.
- Derived parameters (year), which downstream tools require, but that the workflow computes for you.

The workflow can now be run in a few minutes and produce a small compressed CSV file with three columns (date, ZCTA and the climate variable), which is quick to produce and ideal as Bronze-layer input.

Step 4. Adding Database Integration (and Bronze Ingestion)

We now start moving from files on disk to a proper Medallion pipeline.

Dorieh supports ingestion into backends such as PostgreSQL and is gradually adding support for Spark SQL Warehouses. Several tools are available, the most generic being Project Loader that recursively introspects a directory containing data files and creates a database mirroring the directory structure. Consult Dorieh documentation for details on available data loading tools. Here, we will just use the Data Loader Tool to ingest the output of our Climate Pipeline. Using the explicit model definition is best practice (Regulated environments often require explicit data models). Even if not required, explicit models improve collaboration, reproducibility and auditing. In the tutorial we are using PostgreSQL.

The Data Loader Tool (in contrast to the Project Loader that introspects the data and infers the schema) must know the database schema to ingest data. Technically, we can use another Dorieh tool—Introspector to infer the schema from the data file itself (see documentation for Introspector tool), but a good practice (and a requirement in any regulated environment) is to define the schema explicitly via a Data Model Definition in a YAML file. The data model definition language is discussed in Chap. 6 and is described in the Appendix B. We will use the following data model:

Before proceeding we need to:

- Ensure a PostgreSQL database is available.
- Contains Dorieh's core database objects (such as helper functions, internal tables, etc.).
- Connection parameters are identified.

Back in the workflow, we add an input that points to this database configuration file and add an input for which named connection to use.

To support the Medallion architecture and keep Bronze/Silver/Gold tables consistent, versioned and documented we need to explicitly define the data model in Dorieh data-modeling DSL.

The YAML model becomes the single source of truth for:

- Table and view definitions.
- Relationships between layers.
- Transformations and derived fields in higher layers.

In the data model we define a data domain called "tutorial" with a table called "bronze_temperature" specifying at least column names and types and optional descriptions or constraints.

Finally, we add a new workflow step that uses Dorieh Data Loader. The step:

- Depends on the database initialization step, so it only runs after the DB is ready.
- Points to the data model file and the "tutorial" domain.
- Specifies that it should load data into the "bronze_temperature" table.
- Uses the aggregated CSV file from the aggregate step as input.
- Uses the same database configuration and connection name as before.
- Produces logs and error outputs for debugging.

This step takes the output of the file-based pipeline (the per-ZCTA CSV) and converts it into structured rows in the Bronze table. The Bronze Layer now contains "raw" climate data in a normalized tabular shape:

- It is not cleaned or enriched yet.
- But it is structured enough for SQL queries and for building Silver/Gold Layers.

After this step our workflow becomes aware of the database. From now on, downstream transformations are expressed at the data model level (YAML and SQL views/materialized views), rather than as file-level manipulations.

Step 5. Building Medallion Layers (Bronze, Silver, Gold)

It is now time to implement a full Medallion architecture. As discussed in Chaps. 5 and 6, Medallion architecture defines three layers:

- **Bronze Layer**: Load as-is, minimally processed data to database from pipeline outputs.
  - *In this climate data example, the "raw" data is not strictly straight-from-source due to initial aggregation necessary for technical compatibility as NetCDF data cannot be ingested directly into the majority of DBMSs unless a specialized extensions are installed. Hence, we need to transform the data to a more conventional tabular format before ingestion—the exact operation performed by the* **aggregation** *step*
- **Silver Layer**: Clean, harmonize and enrich data.
  - Built from Bronze Layer (no external inputs are allowed).
  - Add derived columns (e.g., Celsius/Fahrenheit conversions, state and city annotation via ZIP lookup).
  - Define as a view on top of the bronze table in your data model YAML.
- **Gold Layer**: Produce analytic/ML-ready outputs.
  - Built from Silver Layer.
  - Perform groupings and summaries (e.g., aggregating by state and date).
  - Use materialized views where performance and reusability are required.

We already have Bronze from Step 4. Now you extend the data model and workflow to include Silver and Gold.

Silver Layer usually is responsible for normalization, harmonization and cleaning of the data as discussed in the Introduction (see the Mad Hatter's Data Preparation Parable section). In our example the data does not require cleansing, as it is already clean, normalized and does not require harmonization because it is coming from a single source. However, even if source data is already clean, enriching it with derived fields or external metadata (such as regional names) increases analytic utility and facilitates downstream ML feature engineering. Hence, we illustrate enriching the data by adding columns, displaying the temperature in different units and annotating ZIP codes with the US State abbreviations and the names of the cities for those areas that lie within a city.

Technically, we

1. Extend the data model:
   - In the same YAML file, define a new object called "silver_temperature":
     - It is declared as a view built from the Bronze table.
     - It includes all three Bronze columns (tmmx, date, zcta).

- It adds new derived columns:
  Temperature in Celsius, computed from the original Kelvin values.
  Temperature in Fahrenheit, computed from Celsius.
  A US state code, computed by looking up the ZCTA and year in a ZIP-to-state mapping function.
  A city name, computed similarly by a ZIP-to-city function.

- These mapping functions rely on reference data that Dorieh manages in the database, installed during the initialization step.

2. Add a Silver-creation step to the workflow:

   - Add a new step (for example, build_silver) that:

     - Depends on the Bronze ingestion step (so Bronze is fully populated first).
     - Uses Dorieh's "create" tool to read the data model.
     - Tells it to create the "silver_temperature" view in the database.
     - Uses the same database configuration and connection.

   - This step also provides logs and errors as outputs.

Because Silver is defined as a database view, it:

- Does not duplicate data; it reads directly from Bronze.
- Can be regenerated at any time from the Bronze data and the current model definition.

From a Medallion perspective, we now have:

- Bronze: "what we ingested".
- Silver: "how we want to see it for general analytics"

After adding the silver layer, we illustrate how to add an analytics/ML-ready Gold Layer. To improve usability for data scientists or analysts this layer aggregates ZCTA daily readings into per-state daily summaries. Similar to Silver Layer it is defined in the data model and built by a create step in the workflow.

Extend the data model with a Gold table:

1. In the YAML data model, define gold_temperature_by_state:

   - It is declared as a materialized view built from Silver.
   - It groups data by two keys:

     - US state.
     - Date.

   - For each state-date combination, it computes:

     - A temperature span (difference between maximum and minimum maximum temperatures across all ZCTAs in the state that day).
     - The mean temperature in Celsius.
     - The mean temperature in Fahrenheit.

- It also defines a primary key on (us_state, date), ensuring each state/day has one row.

2. Add a Gold-creation step to the workflow:

- Add another step (for example, build_gold) that:
  - Depends on the Silver step, so it only runs after Silver is available.
  - Uses the same Dorieh "create" tool and data model file.
  - Instructs it to create the "gold_temperature_by_state" materialized view in the database.

Gold Layer tables are intended for extensive querying, therefore, they use a materialized view rather than a plain view to physically store the aggregated results in the database. This approach improves performance for repeated queries, at the cost of needing refresh logic when underlying data changes.

After running the updated workflow, you should see the following three tables in the database:

1. Table **bronze_temperature** with 3 columns.
2. View (soft) **silver_temperature** with 7 columns.
3. Materialized view **gold_temperature_by_state** with 5 columns.

Looking at the new Gold table, you can observe that:

- The hottest state on that date (January 15, 2019) was Florida, the coldest in the contiguous US was North Dakota.
- The smallest variations of temperature are observed in the smallest states and territories like the District of Columbia, Rhode Island and Delaware and the southern state of Louisiana; the biggest variations are in such geographically diverse states as New Mexico and California.

With a Dorieh pipeline constructed and executed, you are now ready to generate documentation, data dictionaries and column-level lineage—essentials for compliance, collaboration and reproducibility. We cover these next.

Documenting a Workflow

Identifying the Workflow Artefacts You Want to Document

A detailed tutorial on documenting Dorieh workflows is available in the online documentation: https://forome platform.github.io/dorieh/tutorial/climate/documenting-a-workflow.html

The workflow we implemented above is represented by the two YAML files:

- A CWL workflow file that describes **topology and execution** (what steps run and how are they wired?).

- A Dorieh data-model file in Dorieh data-modeling DSL that describes the **logical transformations and schemas** (Bronze/Silver/Gold tables, views and how they are derived).

For documentation, we start from the **process view** (the CWL file) and generate:

- A high-level visualization of the pipeline.
- A machine-readable and human-readable description of its inputs, outputs and steps.

The goal is to produce online, interactive documentation that non-developers (e.g., analysts, reviewers, regulators) can understand without reading raw YAML.

Generating Skeleton Documentation

The goal of this step is to quickly produce a basic, standardized set of docs from the CWL file, which we will then refine. One of the advantages of combining the Common Workflow Language (CWL) with Dorieh data-modeling DSL is the ability to generate meaningful documentation semi-automatically. Dorieh provides the **cwl2md** utility, which transforms a CWL workflow definition file into structured, human-readable Markdown bundle, laying the foundation for reproducibility, transparency and onboarding of new project participants. The output of the utility is illustrated by Fig. 7.1.

The bundle contains a multi-layered documentation artefact:

- **Visual layer**: the DAG diagram shows "how things flow" at a glance.
- **Descriptive layer**: the main Markdown explains inputs, outputs and steps.
- **Source layer**: the CWL source is available in a structured, human-friendly presentation.

At this stage, the docs are largely structural:

- They faithfully describe what the workflow does in terms of parameters and topology.

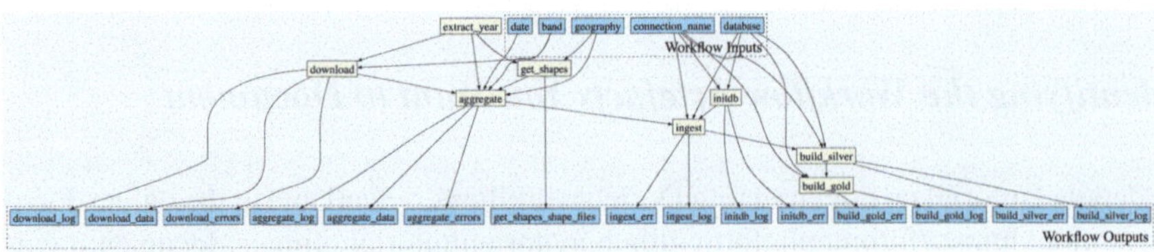

Fig. 7.1 DAG of the example climate workflow

- They may still be light on business context, rationale, or plain-language explanations of why steps exist; all required for effective collaboration and regulatory compliance.

The next steps are about enriching this automatically generated skeleton with additional human-authored narrative, embedded back in the CWL file.

Enhancing Workflow Documentation

First, it is easy to provide a human-readable, high-level title that appears prominently in the generated documentation. The title is embedded in the CWL, binding the documentation to the workflow definition; there is no separate, manually curated doc that can drift out of sync.

Any time cwl2md re-generates docs, it uses this embedded title as the canonical display name.

Next, we turn bare structural metadata into self-explanatory documentation by adding human-written descriptions to inputs, outputs and steps.

The doc field is a first-class documentation channel within CWL that Dorieh's tools understand. They can be included in the definition of the workflow steps, inputs and outputs.

When someone re-runs cwl2md:

- These docstrings are pulled directly into the generated Markdown.
- Inputs, outputs and steps will now show your human-authored text alongside auto-generated structural info.

This has several important effects:

1. **Self-documenting workflows**:
    - Future maintainers (or auditors) do not need to read the raw logic and infer intent.
    - Intent and behavior are explicitly described where they are defined.
2. **Consistency between code and docs**:
    - Because docs live in the same file as the workflow, they are more likely to be updated when the workflow changes.
    - Auto-generation reduces the chance of stale standalone documentation.
3. **Regulatory and collaboration support**:
    - In regulated domains (e.g., healthcare), it is often necessary to show:
        - Exactly what each step is doing.
        - How inputs are interpreted.
        - Where external data or reference mappings come from.

- Using structured doc fields makes it easier to produce documentation that satisfies such requirements without manual rewriting.

Tip: The richer your inline documentation with doc keys and descriptive titles, the more valuable the automated documentation for future users, reviewers and auditors.

Constructing Data Dictionaries and Lineage Graphs

A core requirement for reproducible, auditable research is precise, accessible documentation of all datasets, tables and fields—along with unambiguous tracing of every value's origin. Dorieh provides an integrated dictionary and lineage utility that analyzes your workflow and domain definition file to automatically generate a full suite of human- and machine-readable artefacts: a comprehensive data dictionary and graphical lineage diagrams at both the table and column level.

Start from Your Data Model and Workflow Context

First, we should understand what the dictionary/lineage tool will analyze and why.

The data dictionary and lineage tools treat the data model as the semantic map of the pipeline. By analyzing this model (and optionally the workflow), the tools reconstruct:

- How data flows from one table to another.
- How each column is derived, including intermediate steps.

This is the foundation for generating:

- A data dictionary (human-readable descriptions of domains, tables and columns).
- Lineage diagrams (graphical views of how data moves and transforms).

The Artefacts the Data Dictionary Tool Produces

The following artefacts are produced:

1. Table-level lineage diagram
    - A single graph where each node is a table (e.g., Bronze, Silver, Gold tables).
    - Arrows show dependencies and transformation flow (e.g., Bronze → Silver → Gold).
    - Can be rendered in various image formats such as PNG, SVG, JPEG, etc.
    - In SVG form, each node can be made clickable to open that table's detailed documentation.

2. Table documentation pages
   - One page per table.
   - Contain:
     - Human-readable descriptions pulled from the data model file.
     - The SQL or DDL that defines the table or view.
     - A list of columns with brief metadata and links to column-level pages.
3. Column documentation pages
   - One page per column in every table.
   - Contain:
     - A human-readable description (meaning, units, etc.).
     - A small lineage diagram showing the upstream tables/columns that feed this column.
     - For derived columns, the actual expression or code (often SQL) used to compute it.
     - Clickable nodes/edges in SVG so you can navigate lineage interactively.
4. Global index or glossary of columns
   - A consolidated list of all columns across all tables.
   - Shows where each column appears, how it's reused and in which direction it flows through the medallion layers.
   - Very useful for audits and code reviews when you want to track a particular field across Bronze/Silver/Gold.

Decide Which Formats You Want

A user should know what the tool can produce and how you plan to consume it. Is it going to be used as an internal dev reference? As part of a public or team-wide documentation site? For regulatory or audit purposes? Once you know that, you can pick:

- The right formats (human vs. machine readable).
- The right integration mode (standalone vs. Sphinx).

The output formats are:

- **Markdown** is produced by default, suitable for direct reading or conversion to HTML.
- Additional machine-readable formats like YAML or OBO are available if you need to integrate with external tools (e.g., ontology systems, metadata catalogs).

There are also two operating modes:

- **Standalone mode**:

  - Produces self-contained HTML pages from the generated Markdown.
  - Ideal if you just want a folder to share or archive: open the HTML in any browser and navigate.

- **Sphinx mode**:

  - Adapts the output for integration into a Sphinx + MyST documentation project.
  - Ideal if your lab or team already maintains a Sphinx documentation site and you want the dictionary/lineage to become part of that.

Exploring the Artefacts

The **table-level DAG** gives you a **bird's-eye view**:

- You can quickly see which tables are sources, which are intermediate and which are final analytic outputs.
- The DAG contains **Nodes** (= tables/views) and **Edges** (= "created from" or "depends on") relationships.
- Provides both **visual representation** and cross-linked formal **Documentation pages** in Markdown/HTML.
- You can verify that the Medallion pattern is implemented as intended:

  - **Bronze** → **Silver** → **Gold**, with no unintended shortcuts.

Table pages act as an entry point for **deeper exploration**:

- They combine structural info (schema) and textual explanation.
- They bridge the gap between:

  - Design intent (descriptions and comments).
  - Actual implementation (SQL/DDL).

The **column-level lineage graphs** perform **fine-grained data provenance analysis**. They reveal "which upstream columns contributed to this value?" with the embedded code showing "how exactly was it computed?" and can be used to trace the origin of a specific field from Gold all the way back to Bronze. To construct them, the data dictionary tool:

- Looks at how each derived column is defined (its "source" or expression).
- Finds which upstream tables/columns are referenced.
- Similar to the **table-level DAG**, it provides both **visual representation** and cross-linked formal **documentation pages** in Markdown/HTML.
- **Nodes** represent:

  - Upstream columns and tables that feed into the column.
  - The column itself (as the focal point).

- **Edges** show the **flow of data and transformations**.

- In SVG, nodes/edges are clickable, letting you jump directly to upstream column pages or back to table pages.

A **column documentation page** contains:

- **Metadata header**:
  - The table the column belongs to.
  - The column's fully qualified name (table.column).
  - The data type (e.g., float, integer, text).
  - If provided in the model:
    A human-readable description (meaning, units, semantics).
    A reference URL to external documentation (e.g., a dataset catalog).
- **Compute expression or code** (for derived columns):
  - The SQL or other expression that defines the column as a function of upstream columns.
  - Example: formulas converting from Kelvin to Celsius/Fahrenheit, or aggregations computing means and spans.
- Column-level **lineage diagram**.

To explore, you can:

- Start with the high-level lineage DAG (see Fig. 7.2), where each node is a table.
- **Click** a table to view its documentation, including all columns and their descriptions (Fig. 7.3).
- **Click** on a column name to access its detail page—showing a column-level lineage diagram (Fig. 7.4) for tracing value origins across the workflow.
- All navigation is cross-linked for rapid provenance discovery.

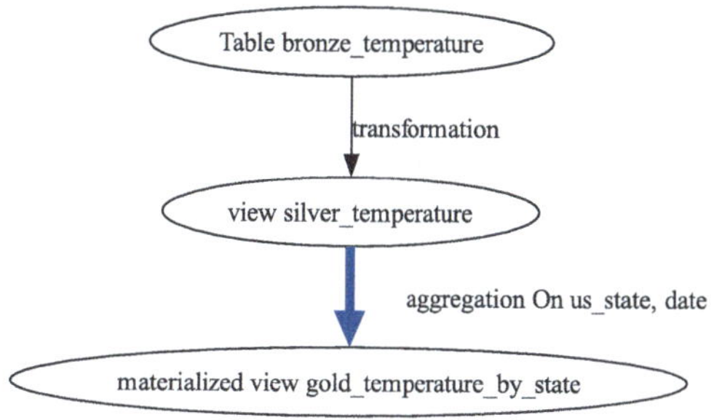

Fig. 7.2 Table-level lineage DAG

Materialized view gold_temperature_by_state

Overview for gold_temperature_by_state

Temperature variations by US State

Aggregated from silver_temperature on On us_state, date

Primary Key: us_state, date

▼SQL/DDL Statement

```
CREATE materialized view  gold_temperature_by_state AS
SELECT
    us_state,
    date,
    MAX(tmmx) - MIN(tmmx) AS t_span,
    AVG(temperature_in_C) AS t_mean_in_C,
    AVG(temperature_in_F) AS t_mean_in_F
FROM silver_temperature

WHERE us_state IS NOT NULL AND date IS NOT NULL
GROUP BY us_state,date;

COMMENT ON materialized view gold_temperature_by_state IS 'CREATED BY Dorieh: {"version": "0.4.3'
```

Columns:

Column Name	Column Type	Datatype
date	grouping	string
t_mean_in_c	computed	float
t_mean_in_f	computed	float
t_span	computed	float
us_state	grouping	string

Fig. 7.3 A screenshot of a gold table description

Making the Documentation Comprehensive

For truly comprehensive documentation some human effort is required. Dorieh data-modeling DSL supports the following keys:

- **description**: a verbose description that explains the element's purpose and semantic meaning
- **reference**: a URL pointing to broader documentation, a project page, or a publication.

For the following elements:

- Domain
- Table
- Column

Additionally, **description** is supported for the Invalid Record element.

The tool pulls all these new descriptions and references into the documentation. The result is a much more **comprehensive data dictionary** that is both:

Column gold_temperature_by_state.t_mean_in_C

Overview of column t_mean_in_C in table gold_temperature_by_state

Table	gold_temperature_by_state
Qualified name	gold_temperature_by_state.t_mean_in_C
Datatype	float
Column type	computed

Mean Temperature in Celsius

Expressions

```
SELECT AVG(temperature_in_C)
```

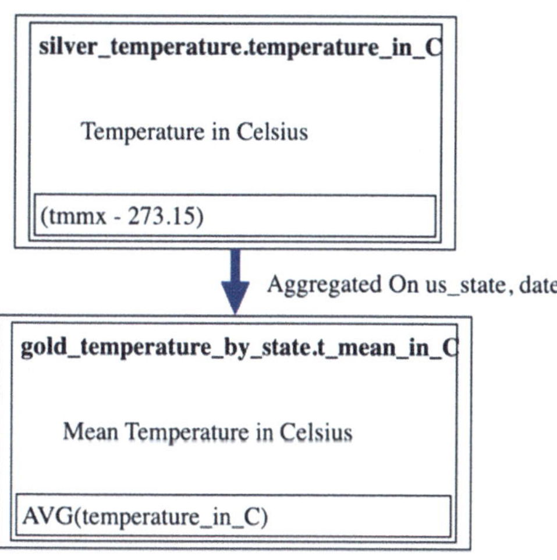

Fig. 7.4 Column lineage DAG and description

- Machine-interpretable (for tooling, validation, search).
- Human-friendly (for analysts, reviewers and domain experts).

Benefits for Compliance, Onboarding and Collaboration

Automated lineage and data dictionary creation are not only best practices for team communication. This level of documentation is not merely nice-to-have: it fundamentally changes how teams, reviewers and regulators engage with your datasets. We believe that these features are critical for satisfying the needs of:

- **Compliance and auditing**: Rapidly answer "Where did this value come from?" or "How is this feature calculated?"—demands familiar to regulated health data, AI model documentation and high-quality science

- **Onboarding and collaboration**: New team members and external collaborators can quickly learn the structure, logic and provenance of your datasets.

Why It Matters

Automated documentation, data dictionaries and interactive lineage:

- Maintain up-to-date, accurate records as pipelines evolve. Documentation always reflects reality (no drift as workflows evolve).
- Accelerate onboarding, audit and publication processes;
- Make reproducible, transparent science the default—rather than the exception.

In the next chapter, we will go to the next level of complexity and illustrate these principles by reviewing and discussing the Dorieh Medicare claims data pipeline, showing how robust provenance and documentation uncover data quality patterns and help address common issues in large, complex datasets.

References

Helena. (2025). *Hexylena/argparse2tool* [Python]. https://github.com/hexylena/argparse2tool (Original work published 2015)

IIDS NKN. (n.d.). Retrieved October 15, 2025, from https://www.iids.uidaho.edu/nkn.php

Chapter 8
Dorieh Medicare Claims Data Pipeline

This chapter uses Medicare claims as a case study to illustrate how the principles of descriptive dataflow operators and provenance-aware workflow design can be applied to complex, longitudinal claims data. Starting from heterogeneous ResDAC source files that vary by year, format and schema, the chapter shows how to design a pipeline that ingests, harmonizes and restructures these inputs into a coherent data warehouse organized into bronze, silver and gold layers. It describes the construction of federated summary and admissions views, the derivation of beneficiaries and enrollments tables and the creation of quality control (QC) aggregates for monitoring data consistency and completeness. The chapter also demonstrates how a data modeling DSL and associated tooling can capture fine-grained data lineage, allowing key variables such as dates of birth and death, residence county and diagnoses to be traced back to their raw sources. While Dorieh is used as an exemplar implementation, the focus is on generally applicable design patterns that support reproducible, provenance-rich claims pipelines under strict privacy and access constraints.

After completing this chapter, readers should be able to:

- Apply the design principles and implementation steps discussed in Chap. 7 to build a provenance-aware pipeline for claims data, from raw ResDAC-style files to analytic-ready tables.
- Explain how raw files from different years and formats can be ingested and harmonized into federated views using a data modeling DSL.
- Distinguish the roles of the key derived structures in a claims warehouse: beneficiaries table, enrollments table and inpatient admissions table.
- Summarize how validation and journaling can be incorporated into an admissions pipeline and how invalid or inconsistent records can be handled without losing auditability.
- Interpret the structure and purpose of QC tables (for enrollments and admissions) and relate them to ongoing data quality monitoring and reporting.

M. Bouzinier et al., *Research Data that Can Be Trusted*,
SpringerBriefs in Computer Science, https://doi.org/10.1007/978-3-032-21032-6_8

- Use table- and column-level lineage diagrams to trace selected claims variables (e.g., DOB, DOD, residence county, diagnoses) from final analytic tables back to heterogeneous raw sources.
- Evaluate how a reproducible, provenance-aware pipeline mitigates common problems when working with restricted claims data, such as duplicated ETL effort, opaque preprocessing and limited shareability of derived datasets.

Processing Health Insurance Claims

Processing health insurance claims is an excellent demonstration use case and a great stress test for a provenance-aware workflow design when building data pipelines. Claims processing pipelines combine many of the hardest problems discussed in earlier chapters: evolving file formats and schemas, large longitudinal volumes, strict privacy constraints and regulatory expectations for reproducibility and auditability. At the same time, claims data is foundational for epidemiology, health services research and environmental health, making the quality and transparency of its preprocessing steps directly relevant to downstream scientific and policy decisions.

In this chapter, we use Medicare claims as a case study to demonstrate how the principles introduced in Parts I and II—descriptive workflow languages, a data modeling DSL, field construction operators and fine-grained lineage—can be applied to a large, heterogeneous claims dataset. The goal is not to teach a specific tool, but to show how a provenance-aware design can be realized in practice under realistic constraints.

We focus on ResDAC Medicare files as an example of a complex input space:

- File formats and schemas differ across years, even for conceptually similar tables such as beneficiary summaries and inpatient admissions.
- Raw data are typically delivered as fixed-width text files accompanied by human-readable "File Transfer Summary" (FTS) documentation, requiring machine-readable schema extraction before ingestion.
- Access conditions are strict: raw files cannot leave accredited environments and preprocessed derivatives cannot be freely shared, leading to repeated "homegrown" pipelines that are rarely documented or reusable.

Within this context, the chapter walks through the design of a claims data warehouse that:

- Ingests raw Medicare files as-is into a bronze layer, preserving original content and structure.
- Harmonizes heterogeneous schemas into federated summary and admissions views, using a data modeling DSL to describe field alignment, transformations and approximations.
- Builds derived beneficiaries and enrollments tables that resolve identity and consolidate longitudinal attributes while explicitly recording ambiguities.

- Applies validation and journaling in the admissions pipeline to separate "bad" records without losing their audit trail.
- Generates quality control (QC) aggregates and lineage diagrams to support systematic monitoring and transparent documentation.

While we use the Dorieh platform as an exemplar implementation, our emphasis throughout the chapter is on design patterns and DSL constructs that can be adapted to other claims datasets and other technical stacks. By the end, readers should see how the abstract concepts of descriptive dataflow operators and provenance-aware workflow design translate into concrete decisions about schemas, validation rules and lineage capture in a realistic Medicare setting.

The text below describes the Medicare Processing Workflow that can be found on Dorieh GitHub (see: https://github.com/ForomePlatform/dorieh/blob/main/src/python/dorieh/cms/models/medicare.yaml and https://github.com/ForomePlatform/dorieh/blob/main/src/cwl/medicare.cwl) documented here: https://forome platform.github.io/dorieh/pipeline/medicare.html

Medicare Claims as a Provenance Use Case

Medicare claims dataset is a canonical example of secondary health data: large-scale, longitudinal and indispensable for research, yet constrained by strong privacy protections and complex data handling agreements, making this domain a perfect setting for examining data provenance and workflow design.

Overview of Medicare/ResDAC Data

In this chapter we discuss handling of the following data categories:

- **Beneficiary (enrollment) files.** Annual "master" files describing each beneficiary's demographic attributes, enrollment status and residence over time, called Master Beneficiary Summary Files (MBSF).
- **Inpatient admissions (claims) files.** Records of hospitalizations, including admission and discharge dates, diagnosis codes and facility characteristics, called MEDPAR files.

These datasets are distributed by the US Government through an agency called *Research Data Assistance Center* (***ResDAC***) as:

- Fixed-width text data files (FWF) and
- Plain-text File Transfer Summary (FTS) documents that describe the layout of the corresponding data file: column names, positions, widths, types and informal descriptions.

From a provenance perspective, several properties are noteworthy:

- **Year-to-year heterogeneity**: Column sets and names change over time. New variables are added; existing variables are renamed; formats evolve. Even logically "the same" table for different years is not schema-identical.
- **Multiple representations of similar concepts**: Beneficiary identifiers, state codes, ZIP codes, dates, and diagnosis fields may appear under different names or slightly different formats across files.
- **Human-oriented metadata**: The FTS documents are written for human readers, not machines. They must be parsed and translated into a formal schema before automated ingestion can occur.

Constraints and Pain Points

Working with Medicare claims under typical data use agreements exposes several recurrent challenges:

- **Restricted access and non-shareable derivatives**. Raw files must remain inside certified environments, and derived tables often cannot be shared outside institutional or contractual boundaries. As a result, different research groups are forced to reconstruct similar preprocessing pipelines independently, with limited ability to review or reuse each other's work.
- **Ad hoc, opaque preprocessing**. Many existing pipelines are composed of scripts and notebooks tied to a particular environment, with limited documentation of assumptions, corrections, or validation steps. Downstream users see only the "final" datasets, with little visibility into how they were constructed.
- **Schema drift over time**. Longitudinal analyses typically span multiple years, but year-specific schema changes are often handled informally (e.g., via hand-written SQL or bespoke scripts). This makes it difficult to reason about, or reproduce, the exact field mappings and transformations that lead to a harmonized analytic table.
- **High stakes for correctness and bias**. Errors in mapping dates, identifiers, residence, or diagnoses can directly affect cohort definitions, exposure assignment and outcome classification. Without documented lineage, it is hard to detect or correct such problems once analytic work has begun.

Why Medicare Is a Strong Provenance Example

The characteristics described above make Medicare claims data a particularly strong test case for the ideas developed in this book:

- It forces us to address **heterogeneous schemas** and **year-to-year evolution** in a principled, declarative way rather than through brittle, one-off code.

- It highlights the need for **fine-grained lineage**: being able to explain, for example, how a given beneficiary's date of birth, date of death, or county of residence in an analytic table was derived from multiple upstream raw records.
- It illustrates why **validation and journaling** are critical. "Bad" records cannot simply be dropped without trace; they must be handled in a way that preserves auditability.
- It shows how a **data modeling DSL** can encode domain knowledge about identifiers, dates, geographic codes and diagnosis arrays in a reusable, portable way.

In the sections that follow, we build on this context to design a claims data warehouse that embodies the principles of descriptive dataflow operators and provenance-aware workflows. We begin with the overall bronze–silver–gold architecture and then examine each stage—raw ingestion, harmonization, derived tables, validation, QC and lineage—in turn.

Designing a Claims Data Warehouse with Bronze–Silver–Gold Layers

The Medicare claims example maps naturally onto the layered Medallion (bronze–silver–gold) architecture discussed in Chap. 5. In this section, we describe how those layers are defined for beneficiary and inpatient admissions data, and how the data modeling DSL is used to make these layers explicit, auditable and reproducible.

Objectives of the Warehouse Design

The warehouse architecture must satisfy several goals simultaneously:

- **Preserve raw inputs** as faithfully as possible, so that transformations are auditable and data flow paths can be followed in both directions.
- **Harmonize heterogeneous schemas** across years without hiding year-specific differences.
- **Provide stable, researcher-friendly analytic structures** (beneficiaries, enrollments, admissions) with clear, documented semantics.
- **Support validation and QC** at well-defined points in the pipeline.
- **Expose lineage** from analytic tables back to raw files at table, column and, when necessary, cell level.

The bronze–silver–gold layering provides a convenient way to organize these requirements.

Bronze: Raw Ingestion and Minimal Conditioning

The bronze layer corresponds to "as-ingested" data that is as close as possible to what ResDAC delivers, while adding just enough structure to make downstream processing manageable.

At this layer:

- Each raw **ResDAC file** (e.g., an MBSF or MEDPAR file for a given year) is ingested into its **own table**.
- The ingestion process uses FTS metadata to parse fixed-width records but does not attempt semantic harmonization.
- A small number of synthetic, uniform columns are added to every table to support cross-file joins and lineage:
  - A field recording the original file name or URI.
  - A record index within the file (see RECORD directive described in Chap. 5).
  - Standardized versions of key identifiers and codes where they can be derived without ambiguity (e.g., a canonical bene_id, year, state, zip column, even if they come from differently named fields upstream).

These tables remain conceptually immutable: new files may be ingested over time, but existing tables are not overwritten in-place. If a file must be re-ingested (for example, due to corrected FTS metadata), this is treated as a new dataset version, preserving the provenance of both.

In the DSL, bronze-layer entities are typically described as **root tables** with columns defined largely by introspected metadata, plus a small number of field construction operators for the synthetic keys.

Silver: Harmonized Views and Longitudinal Structures

The silver layer consists of harmonized, semantically enriched structures built solely from bronze data. No external sources are introduced at this stage. For Medicare, the main silver artefacts are:

- A federated beneficiary summary view that unifies multiple year- and file-specific enrollment tables.
- A federated inpatient admissions view that unifies multiple year- and file-specific claims tables.
- Derived beneficiaries and enrollments tables that resolve beneficiary identity and summarize longitudinal attributes.

At this layer, we introduce more sophisticated field construction operators and aggregations, but we remain careful to:

- Make all transformations **declarative** in the DSL (rather than hidden in ad hoc SQL).
- *Record* **ambiguities and approximations explicitly** (e.g., multiple DOBs for the same beneficiary; county codes inferred from ZIP codes).

In our case, the silver layer includes the following key structures.

Silver: Federated Patient Summary View

The federated patient summary (ps) view combines all enrollment-related bronze tables (e.g., year-specific MBSF files) into a single logical dataset. Its purposes are to:

- Present a uniform set of columns for demographic and enrollment attributes across years.
- Normalize formats for dates, identifiers and codes.
- Provide a stable, queryable basis for downstream aggregation (beneficiaries, enrollments).

The DSL expresses this as:

- A **union transformation** over a set of input tables matching patterns such as cms.mbsf_ab* and cms.mcr_bene_*.
- A set of **field alignment rules** that map year-specific column names (e.g., bene_birth_dt, bene_dob, dob) to canonical fields.
- **Isomorphic transformations** for standardizing representations:
  - Converting two-digit years to four-digit years.
  - Parsing date strings into SQL DATE.
  - Normalizing state and county codes to canonical formats.

The resulting view still reflects the full multiplicity of records—beneficiaries may appear multiple times across years and within a year—but in a schema-coherent way.

Silver: Beneficiaries Table

The **beneficiaries** table is a derived, silver-layer artefact that aggregates the federated summary view to one record per beneficiary. It introduces an explicit **deduplication** and **reconciliation** step.

Conceptually, it performs:

- A **group-by aggregation** on bene_id.
- **Disambiguation rules** for attributes that should have a single value per person:

  - For date of birth (DOB): select the earliest observed value; record the latest as a separate field (dob_latest) when discrepancies exist.
  - For date of death (DOD): select the latest observed value; record the earliest as a separate field (dod_earliest) when discrepancies exist.
  - For race, race (RTI) and sex: aggregate distinct codes into comma-separated lists when multiple values exist.

The DSL expresses these as custom aggregation and disambiguation operators (see Chap. 5 and Part IV). Importantly, the table includes:

- A **duplicates or discrepancy counter** per beneficiary.
- Additional columns carrying the alternative DOB/DOD values when ambiguities are detected.

This design allows analytic users to choose whether to exclude ambiguous beneficiaries and it preserves the information necessary to revisit disambiguation logic later without reingesting raw data.

Silver: Enrollments Table

The enrollments table summarizes, for each beneficiary and year (and often state), enrollment and residence information. It is typically keyed by:

- bene_id
- year
- state (or equivalent territorial key)

Because beneficiaries may move or change addresses within a year, this table must reconcile multiple locations while preserving evidence of heterogeneity. The DSL-driven design:

- Aggregates per-beneficiary-year records from the federated summary view.
- Applies rules to derive:
  - A **canonical state and county of residence** (e.g., selecting one among multiple candidate counties using a deterministic rule).
  - Lists of **all observed states/counties/ZIPs** for that beneficiary-year (e.g., residence_counties, zips).
- Flags:
  - Cases where the county code has been **approximated** (e.g., inferred from ZIP rather than provided directly).
  - Cases where the combination of state, county and ZIP is **internally inconsistent**.

This table also records indicators such as:

- HMO/MAPD enrollment counts.
- Whether the beneficiary died during the year while enrolled.

All of this logic is encoded declaratively in the DSL as combinations of:

- **Rollups** (e.g., from ZIP to county, from county to state).
- **Approximations** (inferring missing geographic codes).
- **Simple and custom aggregates** (e.g., string aggregations of distinct values).
- **Validation flags** attached as additional fields rather than hidden in code.

Silver: Federated Admissions View and Admissions Table

In parallel with the beneficiary-centric structures, the pipeline constructs:

- A **federated admissions view** that unifies all inpatient claims files (e.g., year-specific MEDPAR files), using similar union and field alignment patterns as the patient summary view.
- An **admissions table** that adds:
  - **Normalized** admission and discharge dates.
  - **Standardized** state and ZIP codes for the facility or beneficiary location.
  - **Collapsed diagnosis arrays** from multiple diagnosis columns.
  - Derived attributes such as admission year and hash-based identifiers for approximate distinct counting (e.g., using HyperLogLog).

The admissions table is also the primary focus for validation and journaling, which we discuss in a later section. At the silver layer, the goal is to produce a logically clean, semantically consistent representation of hospitalizations, tied via bene_id to the beneficiaries and enrollments tables.

Gold: Analytic-Ready Aggregates and QC Layers

The gold layer consists of materialized views and tables designed for specific analytic or monitoring purposes. While the silver tables and views contain harmonized and clean data and therefore, to a certain extent can be agnostic to the specific study goals, what data is made available in gold tables is definitely study specific. In our examples, the gold layer includes:

- **QC aggregates**:
  - Enrollment QC tables aggregating beneficiaries by year, state, ZIP and data-quality flags (e.g., consistent vs ambiguous DOB, DOD, race, sex).
  - Admissions QC tables aggregating valid vs invalid admissions by year, state, reason for validation failure and other dimensions.

- **Study-specific analytic tables**, such as:
  - State- or county-level hospitalization counts by year.
  - Cohort-specific views tailored to particular research questions.

Gold-layer artefacts are built exclusively from silver-layer structures, with all transformations expressed via the DSL's dataset and field construction operators. This ensures that:

- **Lineage remains complete**: every value in a gold table can be traced back to silver, bronze and ultimately to specific raw files and record indices.
- **QC tables are reproducible**: their definitions are versioned alongside the rest of the domain definition, avoiding the "spreadsheet trap" where QC logic is lost in manual analyses.

In the remainder of the chapter, we zoom into three aspects of this architecture:

1. How raw ResDAC files and FTS metadata are ingested and harmonized into bronze and silver structures.
2. How validation and journaling are implemented in the admissions pipeline and surfaced through QC tables.
3. How table- and column-level lineage is generated and used to explain derived variables in the Medicare domain.

Raw Ingestion and Schema Harmonization

The first technical challenge in the Medicare pipeline is turning heterogeneous ResDAC files and their human-readable FTS descriptions into a consistent collection of bronze-layer tables and machine-readable schemas. This stage is where we connect the "outside world" of file delivery to the internal world of a data modeling DSL and descriptive workflows.

From FTS Documents to Machine-Readable Schemas

ResDAC delivers each data file (e.g., an MBSF or MEDPAR file for a given year) together with a File Transfer Summary (FTS). An FTS typically includes:

- Column names and brief descriptions
- Physical types (e.g., numeric, character)
- Column positions and widths in the fixed-width file
- Record length and other layout information

To be useful for automated ingestion, this information must be translated into a structured schema that the platform and DSL understand. The general pattern is:

1. **Parse FTS into an intermediate representation**. A parser reads the FTS and extracts, for each column:
   - Name in the raw file
   - Physical type and width
   - Position (start/end offsets)
   - Optional free-text description
2. **Emit a domain definition fragment**. The extracted metadata is serialized into a DSL-compatible format (e.g., YAML) as a table definition with:
   - Column declarations and physical types
   - Optional annotations for descriptions and indexing hints
   - A reference to the input file layout for the ingestion tool
3. **Register the schema**. The resulting domain definition becomes part of the "bronze" layer specification—either as a separate schema file per source, or as part of a consolidated Medicare domain model.

Conceptually, this step is the bridge from human-readable, regulator-oriented documentation to machine-readable, workflow-oriented definitions. It is also where we begin to attach provenance to columns, by associating them with a specific **file**, **year** and layout version.

Ingesting Fixed-Width Files as Bronze Tables

Once the FTS information has been converted into a structured schema, the ingestion process for each ResDAC file follows a predictable pattern:

- **Create a raw table** in the database with one column per FTS-defined field, using physical types compatible with the DBMS (e.g., numeric to INTEGER or NUMERIC, character to TEXT or VARCHAR).
- **Read the fixed-width file row by row**, slicing each line into fields according to the FTS-derived positions and widths.
- **Insert each parsed record** into the corresponding bronze table.

The only transformations applied at this stage are:

- Basic **type coercions** required by the DBMS (e.g., padding or trimming strings, converting numeric strings to integers where unambiguous).
- The addition of synthetic columns to support lineage:
  - A column such as source_file capturing the original file name or URI.
  - A record_index (or equivalent) recording the row number within the file.
  - Optionally, an ingestion timestamp or batch identifier.

These synthetic fields act as the row-level provenance anchors (the equivalent of the FILE and RECORD directives discussed earlier): every downstream value can, in principle, be traced back to a specific file and record index.

Standardizing Key Identifiers and Codes at Ingestion

Some minimal harmonization is necessary already in the bronze layer, to avoid duplicating the same trivial logic throughout the pipeline. In the workflow we are describing, these standardizations are:

- **Beneficiary ID (bene_id)**. Many files use the same identifier but may label it differently. During ingestion, the DSL can define a canonical bene_id column for each table, with a field construction operator that copies from the year-specific name.
- **Year (year)**. The reference year may be provided explicitly or derivable from file naming or metadata. A simple field construction operator can standardize this into an integer year column, ensuring that all bronze tables expose a consistent year dimension.
- **State and ZIP code (state, zip)**. State codes can be standardized into a chosen representation (e.g., FIPS state codes or USPS abbreviations). ZIP codes can be normalized into numeric form and, when nine-digit ZIPs are present, split into base ZIP and ZIP+4 components.

These operations are simple, isomorphic transformations or rollups and are safe to perform at ingestion as long as:

- The original fields are preserved.
- The DSL's domain definition makes all standardizations explicit.

This approach keeps bronze tables close to the raw input while ensuring that a common set of identifiers and geographic keys exist across all sources.

Expressing Bronze Ingestion in the DSL

In the data modeling DSL, bronze tables are typically declared as: **Root tables** within the Medicare domain, each associated with:

- A source file pattern or URI.
- A list of columns derived from FTS metadata.
- Synthetic columns for provenance and standard keys.

Field construction operators at this stage are limited to:

- **Direct copies** (e.g., bene_id from BENE_ID or INTBID).

- **Simple casts and format adjustments** (e.g., trimming, numeric conversion).
- **Derivations from context** (e.g., setting year based on the directory name or file name pattern).

By capturing this logic declaratively, the DSL ensures that:

- The same ingestion rules can be re-applied if files are re-delivered or corrected.
- Alternative backends (e.g., a different DBMS or a Spark-based engine) can implement ingestion consistently from the same high-level specification.
- Downstream lineage tools can see exactly how each bronze column and synthetic field is constructed.

Preparing for Silver: Schema Harmonization Strategy

The final design decision at the raw ingestion stage is how much harmonization to defer to the silver layer. Today, the common best practice is to defer all transformations to the silver layer. However, the described workflow evolved over the years, with initial conception before these best practices have been formulated. Historically, therefore, we adopted a hybrid approach, following this strategy:

- **Bronze layer**: preserve original schema and types, add only cross-cutting keys and provenance anchors.
- **Silver layer**: perform semantic harmonization—unioning tables across years, aligning column names, normalizing dates and codes and introducing higher-level constructs such as beneficiaries and enrollments.

This separation still keeps the bronze layer simple and faithful to the source, while concentrating the more complex, error-prone logic in well-defined silver-level dataset operators. It also aligns with regulatory expectations: bronze tables can be seen as a direct representation of approved ResDAC deliverables, while silver and gold tables are clearly marked as derived artefacts with their own versioned definitions and validation rules.

In the next section, we build on this foundation to describe how the federated views and derived tables in the silver layer are constructed from these bronze ingestions, and how the DSL captures their transformations in a provenance-aware way.

Constructing Silver-Layer Federated Views and Derived Tables

With bronze-layer ingestion in place, the next step is to build harmonized, analytic-friendly structures in the silver layer. In our workflow, these structures are defined declaratively in the domain model (medicare.yaml) and orchestrated via the CWL workflow (medicare.cwl). This section walks through the main silver constructs and highlights how the DSL expresses their transformations and lineage.

Federated Patient Summary View (Ps)

The federated patient summary view is the primary enrollment-centric silver artefact. Its role is to present a single, coherent representation of beneficiary-level attributes across multiple years and legacy file layouts.

Conceptually, the ps view:

- **Unions** multiple bronze tables:
  - All tables whose names match patterns like cms.mbsf_ab* and cms.mcr_bene_ *.
- Applies **field alignment rules** to map heterogeneous column names into a canonical schema:
  - For example, bene_birth_dt, bene_dob and dob all map to a unified dob field.
  - Similar mappings apply to dod, race, sex, address fields, HMO indicators and so on.
- Performs a minimal set of **isomorphic transformations to standardize basic types**:
  - Parsing date fields from character or numeric encodings into SQL DATE types.
  - Converting two-digit years into four-digit years.
  - Normalizing state and county codes into stable logical types (e.g., two-digit FIPS state codes, three-digit SSA county codes).

In the DSL, ps is defined as a view constructed from a set of union transformations and field construction operators. Each canonical field specifies:

- Its type (e.g., date, int, varchar).
- Its sources: one or more upstream columns in the bronze tables.
- The expression implementing its transformation (when needed), expressed either as:
  - A simple cast or function call, or
  - A higher-level operator type (isomorphic transformation, rollup, etc., as classified in Part IV).

Because ps carries the source_file and record_index provenance fields from its bronze inputs, lineage tools can trace any ps record back to the exact file and row from which it was derived.

Beneficiaries Table

The **beneficiaries** table aggregates ps to one row per beneficiary, resolving attribute ambiguities without discarding evidence of inconsistency.

The DSL expresses this table as an aggregation over ps, keyed by **bene_id**, with:

- **Aggregated date fields**:
  - dob: MIN(dob) over all records per bene_id.
  - dob_latest: MAX(dob) over all records; set to NULL when equal to dob.
  - dod: MAX(dod) (latest recorded date of death).
  - dod_earliest: MIN(dod); NULL when equal to dod.
- **Aggregated categorical fields**:
  - race, race_rti, sex: string or array aggregations over distinct values from ps, often implemented as STRING_AGG(DISTINCT …) or equivalent. This allows us to detect and document cases where more than one value has been recorded.
- **Quality indicators**:
  - A duplicates or discrepancies column, counting how many distinct DOB, DOD, race, or sex values were observed.
  - Derived flags such as dob_ambiguous or sex_ambiguous could be introduced as boolean fields generated from these counts.

Within the DSL, these are declared using **custom aggregation operators** and **disambiguation rules**, building directly on the patterns formalized in Part IV ("Aggregations: disambiguation rules"). The DSL structure makes explicit:

- Which attributes are assumed to be single-valued per person.
- How conflicts are resolved (e.g., earliest vs latest, or set-valued representations).
- How ambiguity is surfaced rather than hidden (through supplementary fields).

From a provenance standpoint, the beneficiaries table does not point directly to raw files, but lineage graphs reconstruct the dependency chain through ps, down to the bronze tables and their FILE/RECORD anchors.

Enrollments Table

The **enrollments** table shifts focus from "person across all time" to "person-year (and state)", summarizing where and how a beneficiary was enrolled in a given year. Its primary keys are:

- bene_id
- year

- state (or equivalent territorial key such as state_iso)

The pipeline constructs enrollments as another aggregation over ps (natural-joined with beneficiaries for convenience), with logic including:

- **Residence and geography**:
  - A canonical state and residence_county, often chosen deterministically (e.g., the lexicographically latest among "latest" residence records).
  - fips2 and fips3 codes corresponding to state and county.
  - Arrays or comma-separated lists such as state_list, residence_counties and zips, capturing all observed locations per beneficiary-year.
- **Enrollment continuity**:
  - HMO indicators summarized over the year (e.g., maximum of monthly hmo_indicator values).
  - Count of months with coverage (hmo_cvg_count).
  - A boolean died flag indicating whether the beneficiary died in that year while enrolled in Medicare.
- **Data quality and approximation flags**:
  - state_count: number of distinct states associated with the beneficiary in that year.
  - fips3_is_approximated: true when county FIPS was inferred from ZIP because no valid county code was present in the raw data.
  - fips3_validated: true when the combination of state, county and ZIP passes internal consistency checks.

In the DSL, these fields are described using:

- **Rollup transformations**, mapping detailed geographic codes to broader ones (ZIP → county, county → state).
- **Approximations**, where missing or inconsistent geographic information is repaired in a controlled, documented way.
- **Aggregations** and **array constructions** to collect multiple values and summarize them.
- **Validation-based flags**, added as fields whose values depend on checks over the aggregated record (e.g., comparisons between fips3 and the inferred county from zip).

This design ensures that the enrollments table is both operationally convenient for research (one row per person-year-state) and richly annotated with the decisions and trade-offs made during data harmonization.

Federated Admissions View and Admissions Table

The silver layer also includes constructs focused on hospitalizations:

- A **federated admissions view** (conceptually similar to ps) that unifies all inpatient claims (MEDPAR-like) bronze tables.
- An **admissions table** that normalizes and enriches individual hospitalization episodes.

The federated admissions view is defined in the DSL as:

- A union of all bronze admission tables (e.g., cms.medpar*, cms.mcr_ip_*).
- A set of field alignment rules:
  - Mapping year-specific names for admission date, discharge date, diagnosis codes and facility identifiers into canonical fields.
  - Standardizing date formats to SQL DATE.
  - Normalizing facility location fields (state, ZIP).

The admissions table then adds several layers of derived structure:

- **Temporal fields**:
  - admission_date and discharge_date as normalized dates.
  - admission_year, extracted via a simple isomorphic transformation.
  - Optional fields like admission_day_of_week.
- **Diagnosis representation**:
  - Collapsing multiple diagnosis columns (icd_dgns_cd1, icd_dgns_cd2, …) into a single array field diagnoses, using array construction and flattening operators.
  - Separating primary diagnosis (e.g., pd) from secondary diagnoses, with both stored explicitly and in array form for flexible querying.
- **Approximate distinct counting helpers**:
  - Hash-based fields for bene_id and for diagnoses (e.g., bene_hll, pd_hll, icd_hll), to support HyperLogLog-style approximate COUNT DISTINCT metrics in QC and analytic queries.

All of this is expressed declaratively in the DSL, allowing the same admission-table definition to be compiled into DBMS-specific SQL or, in future implementations, into Spark or other engines. Lineage graphs generated from these definitions clearly show which bronze tables and fields contribute to each element of the admissions table.

Orchestration Via Workflow Definition

While the DSL defines what each silver structure is, the CWL-based workflow defines how and when they are built:

- After bronze ingestion of a given year's files, workflow steps invoke:
  - A "combine tables" or "create view" operation for ps and the federated admissions view.
  - A "create table" operation for beneficiaries, enrollments and admissions, using the DSL definitions as input.
- The workflow expresses dependencies explicitly:
  - beneficiaries and enrollments depend on ps.
  - admissions depends on the federated admissions view and on an initialized database with the necessary functions (e.g., for HLL or ZIP–county mapping).

This separation of concerns—DSL for semantics, workflow for execution topology—aligns directly with the descriptive dataflow operator model introduced earlier: the nodes (dataset operators) are fully specified in the DSL, while the edges and execution order are defined by the workflow engine. The downside though is that due to CWL syntax limitations, these two elements cannot be interlinked and cross-validated. In Appendix B we will explore how this issue can be mitigated with a transition to Groovy-based DSL and integration with nextflow workflow orchestration language.

In the following section, we look more closely at validation and journaling in the admissions pipeline and at how QC aggregates leverage the silver-layer structures to provide a systematic view of data quality across states, years and beneficiary populations.

Validation, Journaling and Quality Control Aggregates

The silver-layer structures described above deliberately preserve as much of the original information as possible, including ambiguities and approximations. The next step is to introduce explicit **validation** and **journaling** so that records that fail well-defined criteria are handled systematically without disappearing from view. On top of this, we build **QC aggregates** in the gold layer to provide an at-a-glance view of data quality.

In our pipeline, these ideas are realized most clearly in the inpatient admissions processing, but the same patterns are general.

Validation of Admissions Data

The admissions table is constructed from the federated admissions view using a dataset operator that also enforces validation rules. These rules are an instance of the three validation types discussed in Chap. 4:

- **Data quality validation** (are individual records internally well-formed?).
- **Validation of algorithms** (does the pipeline behave as specified?).
- **Validation of constraints** (are regulatory or design invariants respected?).

For admissions data, the emphasis is on the first type, with some elements of the second.

In the current implementation, the key checks include:

- **Primary key integrity**.
  - Each admission should have a complete set of key attributes, such as:
    bene_id.
    admission_date.
    discharge_date.
    state or facility location
  - Records with missing or nonsensical values in these fields are flagged as primary-key failures.
- **Referential integrity** with enrollments
  - Every admission must correspond to a beneficiary who is enrolled in Medicare during the year of admission. This is a **foreign key check** against the enrollments table:
    If bene_id, year and state (or other join keys) do not match any enrollment record, the admission is flagged as a **foreign-key failure**.
  - In many cases this indicates either typos in identifiers or inconsistencies between admissions and enrollment files.
- **Duplicate detection.** Identical or near-identical admission records may appear more than once for the same beneficiary. The pipeline detects duplicates based on a chosen key (e.g., bene_id, admission_date, discharge_date, facility ID and primary diagnosis) and:
  - Retains a single "canonical" record in the main admissions table.
  - Labels all other instances as **duplicates**.

These checks are implemented declaratively in the DSL as validation rules associated with the admissions dataset. The rules specify:

- Which fields must be non-null and consistent.
- How to link to the enrollments table for foreign-key checks.
- What constitutes a duplicate.

- What action to take when a rule fails (e.g., "exclude from main table and journal to audit schema").

Journaling Invalid Records

Rather than dropping invalid admissions silently, the pipeline uses a journaling pattern:

- Records that fail any validation check are **not inserted** into the main admissions table.
- Instead, they are written into a dedicated **audit table**, for example medicare_audit.admissions, along with:
  - The reason for failure (e.g., "PRIMARY KEY", "FOREIGN KEY", "DUPLICATE").
  - The full set of fields as they appeared in the federated admissions view.
  - Provenance fields such as source_file and record_index.

This behavior is controlled in the DSL by the dataset's invalid-records policy, as introduced in Chap. 6:

- Default: validation failure aborts the transaction.
- For admissions: override the default to "journal and continue".

This approach has several advantages:

- **Auditability**. All invalid records are preserved and inspectable. Analysts can later review, quantify and potentially correct them.
- **Safety**. Downstream studies built on the main admissions table do not inadvertently include obviously broken records.
- **Transparency**. QC tables and documentation can show, for each year and state, how many admissions were excluded and why.

In a different regulatory or institutional context, the policy could be changed to "fail fast" (abort on first invalid record) or "soft-fail" (retain invalid records but mark them as such). The key is that the policy is explicit, versioned and visible in the domain definition.

Enrollment QC Aggregates

To obtain an overview of data quality for enrollment-related structures, the pipeline defines a QC enrollment materialized view in the gold layer.

Conceptually, this view aggregates over the join of enrollments and beneficiaries, grouped by:

- year
- state
- zip
- fips3 (county)
- Consistency flags derived from the beneficiaries table:
  - consistent_dob (e.g., CONSISTENT, AMBIGUOUS, MISSING)
  - consistent_dod
  - consistent_sex
  - consistent_race
- Approximation and validation flags:
  - fips3_is_approximated
  - fips3_validated

For each group, the view computes measures such as:

- numrecords: the number of enrollment records.
- An approximate numdistinctbeneficiaries, using HyperLogLog summaries (e.g., via a bene_hll field aggregated with hll_union_agg).

In the DSL, this QC table is defined as a materialized view with:

- A group by clause listing all dimensions.
- Aggregation expressions for counts and approximate distinct counts.
- Descriptions for each dimension and measure, which feed directly into the documentation and lineage tools.

This QC artefact allows analysts to:

- Inspect, for any year and region, how many beneficiaries have ambiguous DOB, DOD, race, or sex.
- Examine where geographic approximations (e.g., county inferred from ZIP) are most prevalent.
- Monitor changes in data quality over time or across states.

Admissions QC Aggregates

A parallel QC table is defined for admissions, aggregating both valid and invalid records:

- The main admissions table and the audit table medicare_audit.admissions are combined (for example, via UNION ALL) into a logical input.
- The QC view groups by:
  - year
  - state
  - zip

  - reason (with values such as OK, PRIMARY KEY, FOREIGN KEY, DUPLICATE)

- For each group, it computes:
  - numrecords: total admissions (including those failed validation).
  - numdistinctbeneficiaries: approximate distinct count of beneficiaries using bene_hll.

From these base measures, additional metrics can be defined in analytic tools (e.g., BI dashboards) as percentages:

- Percent of valid admissions (reason = 'OK').
- Percent of admissions with missing key data (reason = 'PRIMARY KEY').
- Percent of admissions with enrollment mismatches (reason = 'FOREIGN KEY').
- Percent of duplicate admissions (reason = 'DUPLICATE').

Again, the DSL describes the QC table as a materialized view with explicit grouping dimensions and measures. This makes the QC definitions:

- Version-controlled alongside the rest of the domain model.
- Consistent across environments (development, testing, production).
- Inspectable by lineage and documentation tools.

Role of QC in a Provenance-Aware Pipeline

QC aggregates serve two roles in a provenance-aware design:

- **Operational monitoring**. They provide a quick, quantitative summary of data quality issues across time and geography. This helps teams prioritize remediation, understand limitations of the data for specific research questions and support internal governance.
- **Evidence for reproducibility and compliance**. Because QC tables are defined declaratively in the DSL and built from the same silver structures as analytic tables, they become part of the documented processing chain. When publishing findings or responding to audits, researchers can point to:
  - The exact QC definitions.
  - The distributions of validation failures.
  - The proportion of data excluded for specific reasons.

Under the hood, QC tables are simply another instance of dataset operators in the DSL, using aggregations and rollups over the core tables. Their significance lies in the way they surface the "health" of the pipeline itself.

In the next section, we turn to data lineage: how table- and column-level lineage diagrams are generated from the Medicare domain definition, and how they can be used to trace specific variables (like residence county or primary diagnosis) from gold-layer tables all the way back to the raw ResDAC files and record indices.

Data Lineage and Documentation in the Medicare Pipeline

In the Medicare pipeline, lineage and documentation are not additional afterthoughts but a direct consequence of how the domain is modeled in the DSL. Because every dataset operator and field construction operator is declared there, the same information can be reused to generate table- and column-level lineage views and a data dictionary for the entire Medicare domain.

Table-Level Lineage: The Medicare DAG

At the table level, the Medicare domain definition yields an informative DAG (see Fig. 8.1) containing:

- **Bronze**: one table per ResDAC file (e.g., cms.mbsf_abcd_2018, cms.medpar_2018), plus synthetic FILE/RECORD fields.
- **Silver**:
  - ps (federated patient summary) from all MBSF-like tables.
  - Federated admissions view from all MEDPAR-like tables.
  - beneficiaries and enrollments from ps.
  - admissions from the federated admissions view, with referential checks to enrollments.
- **Gold**:
  - Enrollment and admissions QC tables from the silver tables and the audit schema.
  - Any study-specific aggregates from enrollments and admissions.

The generated table-level lineage diagram makes this structure visually explicit. For a reviewer, it answers quickly:

- Which upstream raw files contribute to a given analytic or QC table?
- Where in the pipeline are unioning, aggregation, or validation applied?
- Which tables depend (even indirectly) on approximations such as ZIP→county mapping?

Because this DAG is derived from the same YAML that defines the datasets, it stays in sync as the domain evolves.

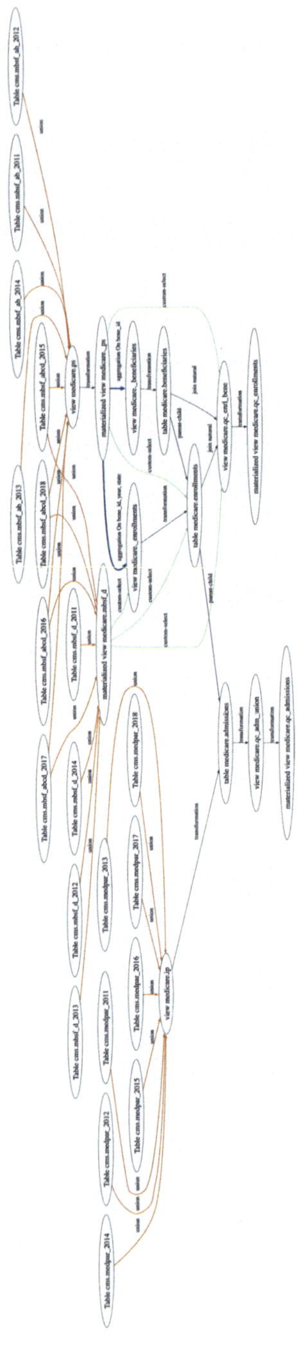

Fig. 8.1 Medicare Table Lineage

Column-Level Lineage: Two Illustrative Variables

Column-level lineage is often where provenance becomes most practically useful. In the Medicare pipeline, two fields illustrate this: date of birth (DOB) and residence county.

DOB in the Beneficiaries Table

The DSL for beneficiaries specifies that:

- dob is MIN(dob) over all ps records for a given bene_id.
- dob_latest is MAX(dob), set to NULL when equal to dob.
- A discrepancy count (or equivalent) is also computed.

Column-level lineage for beneficiaries.dob (See Figs. 8.2 and 8.3) shows that:

- It is an aggregation over ps.dob.
- ps.dob in turn is built from one or more upstream columns per year (e.g., bene_birth_dt, bene_dob), each parsed and normalized.
- Those upstream columns originate in specific bronze tables tied to concrete ResDAC files and FTS entries.

From a single lineage diagram, a reader can see both the rule ("earliest DOB wins, latest is kept separately") and the sources (which raw fields and years feed into that decision). This is precisely the level of detail often needed in methods sections, internal reviews, or regulatory documentation.

Residence County in the Enrollments Table

For residence_county (or its corresponding FIPS code), the DSL encodes:

- Whether the county value came directly from a raw county field or was approximated from ZIP.
- How multiple locations within a year are reduced to a canonical value (e.g., deterministic selection plus a list of all observed counties).
- Consistency checks between state, county and ZIP.

The column-level lineage graph (see Fig. 8.4) for enrollments.residence_county therefore shows:

- The rollup and approximation operators involved.
- Any joins to reference geography tables (if used).
- The ultimate origin of the input ZIP and county codes in the bronze MBSF tables.

This makes it straightforward to answer questions like: "For this analysis, did you ever infer counties from ZIP codes? If so, where?"

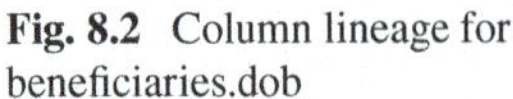

Fig. 8.2 Column lineage for beneficiaries.dob

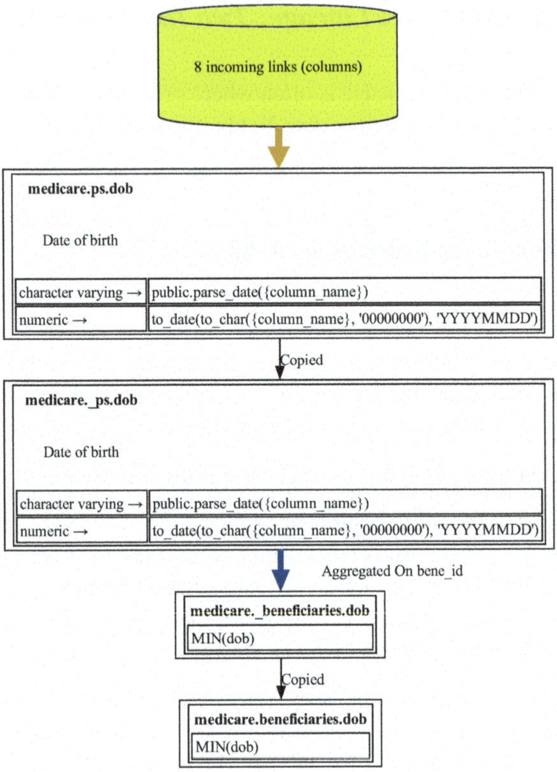

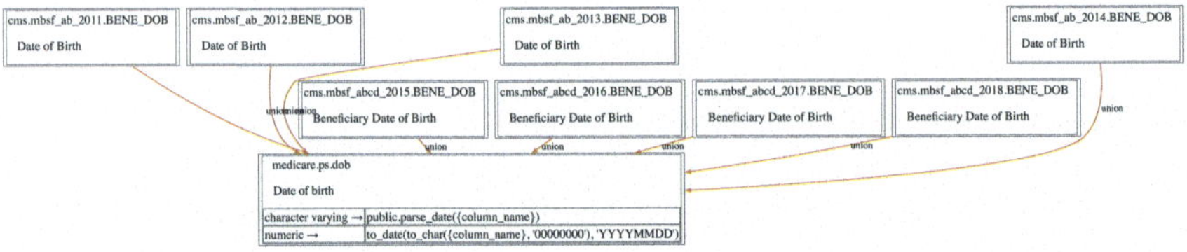

8 incoming links (columns)

medicare.ps.dob

Date of birth

character varying → public.parse_date({column_name})

numeric → to_date(to_char({column_name}, '00000000'), 'YYYYMMDD')

Copied

medicare._ps.dob

Date of birth

character varying → public.parse_date({column_name})

numeric → to_date(to_char({column_name}, '00000000'), 'YYYYMMDD')

Aggregated On bene_id

medicare._beneficiaries.dob

MIN(dob)

Copied

medicare.beneficiaries.dob

MIN(dob)

cms.mbsf_ab_2011.BENE_DOB Date of Birth

cms.mbsf_ab_2012.BENE_DOB Date of Birth

cms.mbsf_ab_2013.BENE_DOB Date of Birth

cms.mbsf_ab_2014.BENE_DOB Date of Birth

cms.mbsf_abcd_2015.BENE_DOB Beneficiary Date of Birth

cms.mbsf_abcd_2016.BENE_DOB Beneficiary Date of Birth

cms.mbsf_abcd_2017.BENE_DOB Beneficiary Date of Birth

cms.mbsf_abcd_2018.BENE_DOB Beneficiary Date of Birth

union

medicare.ps.dob

Date of birth

character varying → public.parse_date({column_name})

numeric → to_date(to_char({column_name}, '00000000'), 'YYYYMMDD')

Fig. 8.3 Column lineage for ps.dob

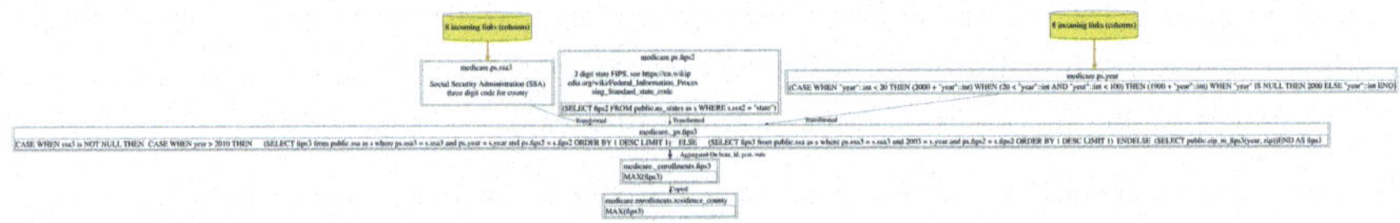

Fig. 8.4 Column lineage for residence_county

How Users Consume Lineage and Documentation

Because the same DSL drives both execution and documentation, the pipeline can automatically provide:

- **HTML/Markdown pages per table and per column**, with:
  - Descriptions, types and SQL/DDL snippets.
  - Links into lineage diagrams.
- **Interactive lineage diagrams** (typically SVG):
  - A global table-level view.
  - Column-specific views highlighting contributing upstream fields.

Analysts and reviewers typically use these artefacts in two ways:

- **Top-down**: Starting from a gold-layer field (e.g., "number of admissions with consistent DOB in 2018, by state"), they follow links back through QC tables, admissions, enrollments and ps to see exactly how the measure is constructed.
- **Bottom-up**: Starting from a raw field in a specific ResDAC file, they explore how and where that field is used downstream and whether any approximations or disambiguation rules apply.

In the Medicare pipeline, this closes the loop: every analytic feature or QC metric is not only computed reproducibly, but also explainable in terms of concrete upstream files, fields and operators—without manual reverse-engineering.

QC Results: Quality of Medicare Data

The Medicare pipeline described in this chapter, together with its DSL-defined QC aggregates, allows us to quantify the prevalence and structure of inconsistencies in both beneficiary-level and admission-level data.

The results summarized below are based on seven years of data (2011–2014 and 2016–2018) and have been presented at the Intelligent Systems for Molecular Biology Conference (Audirac et al. 2023). Although this is not the full temporal span of Medicare, it is long enough to reveal stable patterns and to illustrate how a provenance-aware design supports data quality assessment.

Consistency of Beneficiary Data

Across approximately 80 million unique beneficiaries observed over the seven-year window, 99.33% of records are internally consistent with respect to the core demographic attributes tracked in the beneficiaries table (date of birth, date of death, sex

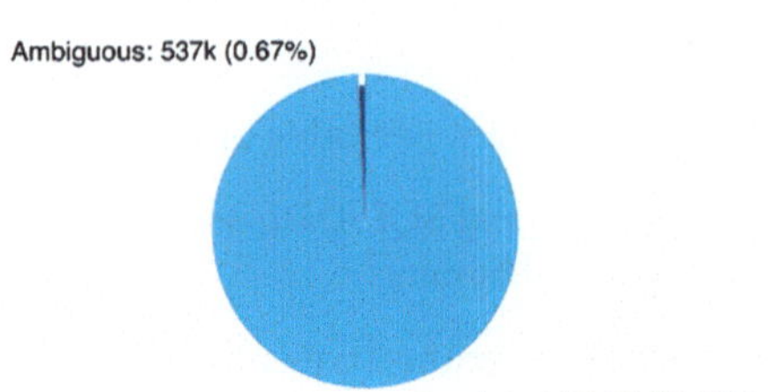

Fig. 8.5 Discrepancies in Medicare enrollments data

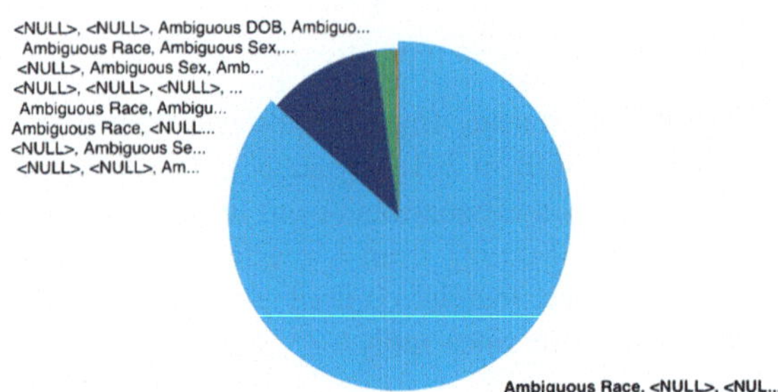

Fig. 8.6 Types of discrepancies in Medicare enrollments data

and race). Only 0.67% of beneficiaries exhibit any discrepancy across years in one or more of these fields (see Figs. 8.5 and 8.6).

Decomposing this 0.67% reveals that:

- **Race** is the dominant source of inconsistency, accounting for roughly 85% of all discrepant beneficiaries. This is not surprising: race is self-reported, may change over a lifetime and is particularly prone to variation for people with mixed or evolving identities. It is also sensitive to changes in coding practices and data collection instruments over time.
- **Date of birth (DOB)** differences contribute about 11% of all inconsistencies. These are examined in more detail in the next subsection.
- **Sex** inconsistencies account for slightly under 2% of discrepant beneficiaries. While numerically small, such discrepancies can be important in specific research contexts (e.g., sex-stratified analyses).
- **Date of death (DOD)** is rarely ambiguous: only about 0.05% of beneficiaries (roughly 250 individuals in this sample) exhibit multiple, conflicting death dates across enrollment records.

Two points are worth emphasizing from a provenance perspective:

- The beneficiaries table does not silently "fix" these issues. Instead, it records both reconciled values (e.g., earliest and latest DOB, latest DOD) and **explicit**

flags and counts of distinct values, enabling downstream users to either filter out ambiguous beneficiaries or perform sensitivity analyses.
- Because the reconciliation rules and aggregation operators are defined declaratively in the DSL, the consistency metrics themselves are reproducible: re-running the pipeline on updated data or in another environment will yield the same classification of consistent vs inconsistent records.

The QC aggregates discussed earlier summarize these patterns at the level of year and geography, but the underlying information is available down to individual beneficiaries via the silver-layer tables.

Errors in Date of Birth (DOB)

Ambiguous dates of birth provide a concrete example of how provenance-aware aggregation and QC reveal the structure of data errors.

In our seven-year sample, approximately **60,000 beneficiaries** have more than one recorded DOB in the federated patient summary (ps) and thus are classified as having ambiguous DOB in the beneficiaries table. However, the distribution of DOB discrepancies suggests that most of these are minor clerical issues rather than fundamentally conflicting information.

Key observations include:

- The largest single group—about **20,600** beneficiaries have DOB values that differ by exactly **one day** across records. Another roughly **20,000** beneficiaries have discrepancies of **less than a week**. These small offsets are plausibly attributable to transcription errors, or minor inconsistencies in original paperwork. For many analytic purposes (especially studies insensitive to a few days' age difference), such discrepancies may be ignorable.
- Beyond these small differences, the histogram (see Figs. 8.7 and 8.8) of absolute DOB differences shows distinct peaks at:
  - Exactly 10 days,
  - Approximately 20 days,
  - Roughly one, two and three months and
  - Exactly one year, two years and higher integer year offsets.

These peaks strongly suggest typical typographical patterns, such as:

- A single digit mistyped in the day or month.
- A shift of the month by ± 1 or $\pm$ 2.
- A year mis-keyed by ± 1 or $\pm$ 10 (e.g., "1949" vs. "1959").

From the point of view of the beneficiaries table:

- The reconciliation rule (earliest vs latest DOB) is transparent and deterministic, and both values are retained when they differ.

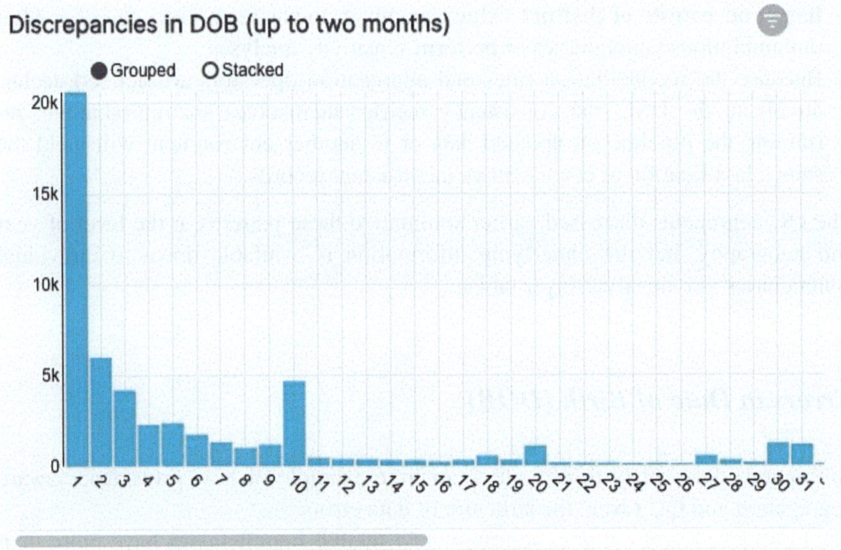

Fig. 8.7 Discrepancies in the Date of Birth (less than 30 days)

- An analyst who cares about fine-grained age (e.g., pediatric or near-threshold age studies) can use the discrepancy measures to exclude ambiguous DOBs or to conduct sensitivity analyses.
- For many adult cohorts where only age in whole years matters, it may be sufficient to either accept the reconciled DOB or apply additional study-specific heuristics (for example, excluding cases with differences exceeding one month or one year).

The key enabling factor is that the DSL encodes both the reconciliation logic and the aggregation used to construct discrepancy statistics, making it straightforward to regenerate histograms and to refine rules without re-writing low-level code.

Discrepancies in Inpatient Admission Data

The admissions pipeline introduces validation and journaling to classify hospitalization records into valid admissions and several categories of "bad" data (see Figs. 8.9 and 8.10). Here, too, systematic QC aggregates reveal the dominant failure modes and their geographic distribution.

At the national level, three patterns stand out:

- **Missing core fields** are the primary cause of invalid admissions. These include missing beneficiary identifiers, missing or non-parsable admission or discharge dates and other fields required to form a valid primary key. Records failing these

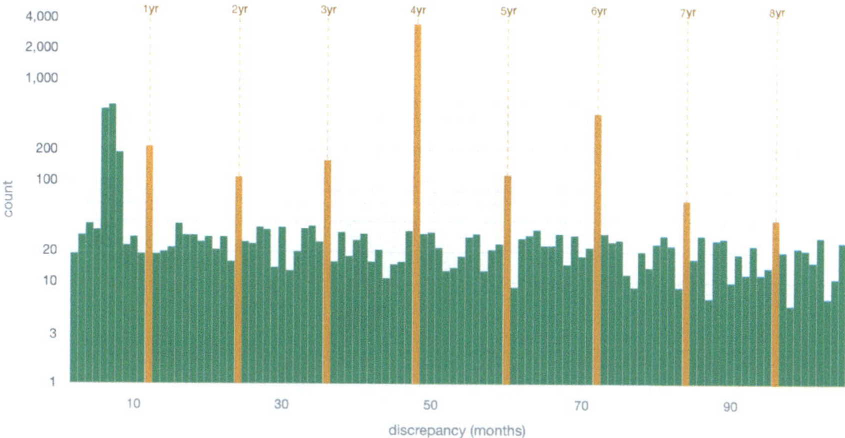

Fig. 8.8 Discrepancies in the Date of Birth (more than 30 days)

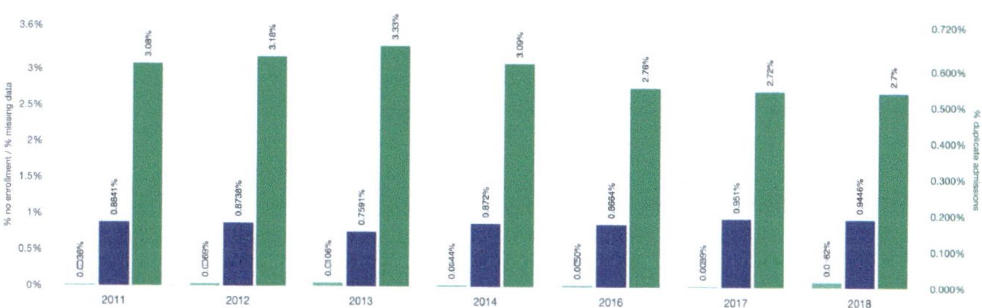

Fig. 8.9 Admissions failing validation by year

checks are excluded from the main admissions table and written to the audit table with reason codes such as PRIMARY KEY or MISSING.

- **Admissions without matching enrollment** form the second largest error category. These are hospitalizations for which no corresponding beneficiary-year record exists in the enrollments table, according to the defined join keys (bene_id, year and sometimes state). In many cases, this likely reflects errors in beneficiary identifiers or misalignments between admissions and enrollment files. In our QC tables, these records are grouped under a reason such as FOREIGN KEY.
- **Duplicate admissions** exist but are relatively rare compared to the other two categories. When duplicates are detected by the pipeline's duplicate key rules, one admission is retained as canonical in the main table, and the others are journaled with a reason such as DUPLICATE.

The QC aggregates further break down these issues by state, revealing marked spatial variation:

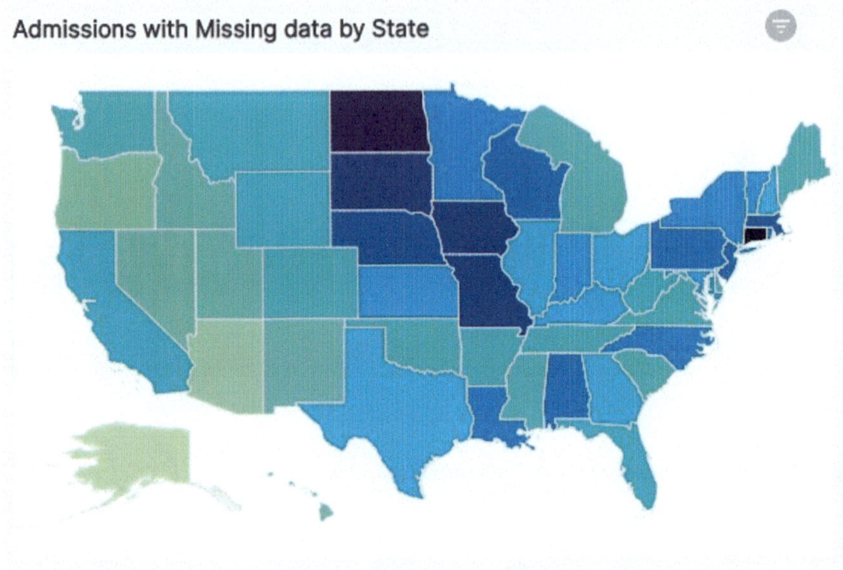

Fig. 8.10 Admissions failing validation by State

- The rate of **admissions with missing data** (e.g., missing key fields) is highest in North Dakota and Connecticut, followed by Massachusetts and several Midwestern states. At the other end of the spectrum, Alaska, Oregon, and Arizona exhibit relatively low rates of missing-data admissions.
- **Duplicate admissions** are few in absolute terms and appear relatively evenly distributed across states, making detailed spatial patterning harder to interpret.
- **Admissions without matching enrollment** display a distinct geographic pattern:
  - Nevada stands out as a clear outlier with the highest proportion of such records, followed by Alaska, Arizona and Wyoming.
  - The lowest rates of admissions lacking enrollment matches are observed in several Midwestern states, Massachusetts and California.

These findings underscore two broader points:

- **Validation rules have interpretable signatures**. Because the criteria for classifying records as PRIMARY KEY, FOREIGN KEY, or DUPLICATE are explicitly defined in the DSL, differences in error rates across states and years can be investigated in a principled way—by examining upstream files, coding practices and local data-entry conventions.
- **Journaling preserves the evidence**. None of the "bad" admissions disappear; they are systematically recorded with reason codes and provenance fields. This allows future investigators to:

- Revisit the validation thresholds (e.g., accept some previously excluded records in sensitivity analyses).
- Trace problematic patterns (such as unusually high FOREIGN KEY failures in a given state and year) back to specific raw files and even individual records.

Taken together, the beneficiary-level and admission-level quality assessments illustrate the practical value of a provenance-aware pipeline: it not only produces analytic-ready tables, but also generates a rich, reproducible picture of the strengths and limitations of the underlying data. This, in turn, supports more nuanced study design, more transparent reporting of data quality and more informed conversations with data providers and regulators about potential remediation or improvement of source datasets.

Reference

Audirac, M., Bouzinier, M., Braun, D., Shad, M. M., & Yockel, S. (2023). Systematic approach to preparing of medical claims data for biomedical research. *F1000Research, 12*. https://doi.org/10.7490/f1000research.1119612.1

Chapter 9
What Is Next?

This chapter discusses the development and implications of using Domain-Specific Languages (DSLs) for data provenance, emphasizing ethics and compliance with complex regulations such as EHDS, AI Act and HIPAA. The Dorieh Data Platform demonstrates the practical application of these concepts. It highlights the importance of expressive DSLs for capturing detailed data transformations and ensuring compliance and transparency. Future directions include evolving Dorieh to integrate with existing metadata standards like Croissant-RAI and exploring productization opportunities to support broader adoption and impact in data governance.

After completing this chapter, readers will be able to:

1. Evaluate emerging trends in data provenance and DSLs
2. Assess the integration potential with existing metadata standards
3. Plan for future developments in compliance requirements
4. Identify opportunities for data platform enhancement
5. Discuss appropriate productization strategies

Ethics and Multimodal Regulation in Data Provenance

Our work on Domain-Specific Languages (DSLs) for data transformation and provenance tracking originated from the need to ensure reproducibility and accountability in data-intensive research. Conducted within the controlled environment of the Harvard University Faculty of Arts and Science Research Computing (FASRC), we utilized research datasets from the Centers for Medicare & Medicaid Services (CMS) to address challenges in documenting and reproducing complex data preprocessing workflows. However, the techniques and tools developed in this controlled setting are adaptable to less controlled environments, such as the emerging European Health Data Space (EHDS) ecosystem, which must navigate diverse national and international laws and a plethora of use cases across geographies.

M. Bouzinier et al., *Research Data that Can Be Trusted*,
SpringerBriefs in Computer Science, https://doi.org/10.1007/978-3-032-21032-6_9

Multimodal regulation refers to the simultaneous compliance with overlapping and sometimes conflicting regulatory and governance frameworks, examined in detail in Part III. These frameworks demand data quality, security, transparency and ethical accountability. Our DSL approach inherently supports these dimensions by embedding provenance tracking directly into workflows, enabling detailed documentation of data transformations, validation steps and lineage. For instance, the lineage tracking mechanisms developed for Medicare datasets provide clear, auditable records that align seamlessly with the transparency mandates of the EHDS and the risk assessment requirements of the AI Act.

The scalability of our tools lies in their ability to address ethical and regulatory concerns in diverse environments. In curated settings like Medicare data analysis, the provenance techniques ensure reproducibility and fairness by validating transformations and minimizing biases. In broader ecosystems like the EHDS, these tools can adapt to more heterogeneous datasets and dynamic compliance needs, providing a robust foundation for transparency and accountability across borders.

Looking ahead, the application of these provenance tools to multimodal regulation represents a promising direction for creating unified compliance strategies. By leveraging curated datasets to refine methodologies, organizations can scale these approaches to address emerging challenges in AI ethics, data governance and cross-border collaboration.

Future Directions for Provenance Tools

As the regulatory and technological landscape evolves, provenance systems must advance to meet new demands for transparency, scalability and community adoption. Two critical areas of focus are transitioning to more expressive DSL implementations and ensuring project sustainability.

Transitioning to Expressive DSLs

While our current YAML-based DSL provides a strong foundation for documenting data provenance, several areas require further development to support the increasing complexity of regulatory and operational environments. Transitioning to a more expressive DSL, potentially based on Apache Groovy, offers significant advantages. Groovy's flexibility and readability make it well-suited for capturing complex data transformations, enabling researchers to document workflows more effectively while maintaining accessibility. Appendix B describes Dorieh current approach to transitioning to Groovy-based DSL.

This evolution aligns with the growing documentation requirements for AI systems under frameworks like the EU AI Act, where transparency and traceability are paramount. An expressive DSL can facilitate the seamless integration of provenance documentation into diverse workflows, ensuring that organizations can meet evolving compliance demands without compromising usability. In Part III we will elaborate on these ideas.

Ensuring Project Sustainability

Building a sustainable community around provenance tools is essential for long-term success. This includes fostering a user base that can contribute to the platform's development while maintaining the rigorous documentation capabilities needed for regulatory compliance. Key strategies include:

- **Enhancing Usability**: Simplifying the tools to ensure they are accessible to both technical and non-technical users.
- **Encouraging Collaboration**: Supporting an open ecosystem where researchers, developers and regulators can contribute and share best practices.
- **Supporting Scalability**: Ensuring that the tools can handle diverse datasets and regulatory requirements across different domains and geographies.

Our work with DSLs and data provenance tracking points toward a promising future for responsible data governance. By building on the lessons learned from Medicare data analysis and adapting to the demands of less controlled environments, provenance tools can become a cornerstone of modern compliance strategies. This approach aligns with the principles of transparency, accountability and adaptability, ensuring that data-driven systems remain ethical, compliant and reliable.

Potential for Integration with Workflow Definition DSLs

Nextflow uses a Groovy-based DSL to define topology, inputs, requirements and outputs of a computational workflow, e.g., a workflow required for the ETL process. If a data modeling DSL is also Groovy-based it creates a potential for integration of the whole ETL process into a single uniform library of Groovy-based scripts. For a potential example of defining a data model using a Groovy-based DSL see Appendix B.

We should note that the current Dorieh, YAML-based DSL is logically compatible with CWL—also a YAML-based DSL for workflow topology definition. However YAML files are less flexible hence it is more difficult to organize them as a uniform library.

Spark Implementations

Dorieh currently implements the data modeling DSL by compiling it into a set of SQL statements for PostgreSQL. It seems attractive to also add an Apache Spark (Zaharia et al. n.d.) based implementation, when the DSL expressions are compiled into Scala or Python code for Spark. Spark tables are represented as Parquet files, ordinary files on a file system. Dorieh already has built-in export to Parquet, including an option to make exported files Spark-compatible.

One of the advantages of the Spark implementation would be its serverless nature. PostgreSQL requires a running server. While to take advantage of all Spark features, HDFS (*HDFS Architecture Guide* n.d.) and a dedicated Spark auto-scaling infrastructure are required, a simple Spark program can be run on any compute node with Java Virtual Machine (JVM).

Advancing Compliance through Machine-Readable Dataset Documentation

The work by Jain et al. (2024) on Croissant-RAI introduces a comprehensive framework for responsible AI (RAI) documentation, emphasizing structured metadata to improve dataset discoverability, interoperability and trustworthiness. While Croissant-RAI focuses on AI datasets, its principles provide a strong foundation for advancing data provenance practices across domains where provenance is critical, such as healthcare and clinical research regulated globally as presented in Part III.

A key feature of Croissant-RAI is its structured properties, such as *rai:dataCollectionMissingData*, *rai:dataPreprocessingProtocol* and *rai:dataAnnotationAnalysis*, which capture various aspects of data quality and processing. These properties are currently represented as free-text (*src:Text*), which limits their utility for automation and machine-driven validation. Transitioning these properties into a Domain-Specific Language (DSL) format enables structured, machine-readable documentation, facilitating automation, reproducibility and compliance.

In the context of data provenance, a DSL approach provides significant advantages. For example:

- Enhanced Lineage Tracking: Properties like *rai:dataPreprocessingProtocol* can precisely describe transformations applied to datasets, enabling traceability from raw inputs to final outputs.
- Regulatory Alignment: By structuring metadata in a DSL, organizations can ensure their documentation meets specific requirements of frameworks like those reviewed in Part III, which demands clear documentation of data handling processes.

- Interoperability Across Jurisdictions: DSL-based documentation supports dynamic rule composition, allowing organizations to adapt metadata templates to the varying requirements of different regulatory environments.

By generalizing Croissant-RAI's methodologies, data provenance can move beyond AI-specific use cases to address broader challenges in healthcare and other data-intensive fields. This structured approach enables organizations to encode provenance information directly into workflows, ensuring transparency, accountability and compliance while maintaining the flexibility to adapt to evolving regulatory landscapes.

In conclusion, the adoption of DSLs for documenting data provenance represents a critical evolution in responsible data governance. By building on frameworks like Croissant-RAI, organizations can achieve a unified, scalable approach to metadata management, enhancing both compliance and the trustworthiness of data-driven systems.

Productization Potential

Looking forward, the evolution of Dorieh and its DSL into a more expressive implementation, potentially based on Apache Groovy, represents an exciting opportunity. This transition will enhance the platform's capability to document complex transformations while maintaining usability for researchers and compliance professionals. Furthermore, the potential productization of Dorieh offers a route to broader adoption and impact. By evolving Dorieh into a market-ready solution, the platform can support a wide range of stakeholders, including healthcare providers, researchers and regulatory agencies, enabling them to integrate provenance tracking seamlessly into their data governance workflows.

Productization would involve not only refining the platform's technical capabilities but also ensuring its scalability, accessibility and alignment with industry standards. Key steps could include:

- **Commercialization**: Investigate the market potential within established product categories such as Trusted Research Environments and Secure Processing Environments. Develop a roadmap for evolving the platform to address emerging needs outside its existing use cases. This includes identifying new stakeholder groups, such as international regulatory bodies or cross-sector industries and tailoring Dorieh to serve diverse compliance and operational requirements.
- **Building a Robust Ecosystem**: Foster partnerships with regulatory bodies, academic institutions and industry players to ensure the platform meets global compliance and operational needs.
- **Developing Modular Features**: Offer customizable modules tailored to specific regulatory frameworks or domains, enabling flexibility and ease of integration.

- **Promoting Open Standards**: Ensure interoperability with existing systems and standards, such as Health DCAT-AP (*Health DCAT-AP Specification*, n.d.) and Croissant-RAI, to maximize adoption and usability.

References

HDFS Architecture Guide. (n.d.). Retrieved October 31, 2024, from https://hadoop.apache.org/docs/r1.2.1/hdfs_design.html

Health DCAT-AP Specification. (n.d.). Retrieved December 25, 2025, from https://healthdcat-ap.github.io/

Jain, N., Akhtar, M., Giner-Miguelez, J., Shinde, R., Vanschoren, J., Vogler, S., Goswami, S., Rao, Y., Santos, T., Oala, L., Karamousadakis, M., Maskey, M., Marcenac, P., Conforti, C., Kuchnik, M., Aroyo, L., Benjelloun, O., & Simperl, E. (2024). *A Standardized Machine-readable Dataset Documentation Format for Responsible AI* (No. arXiv:2407.16883). arXiv. https://doi.org/10.48550/arXiv.2407.16883

Zaharia, M., Chowdhury, M., Franklin, M. J., Shenker, S., & Stoica, I. (n.d.). *Spark: Cluster Computing with Working Sets*.

Part III
The Architecture of Trust: Regulation, Provenance and Compliance-as-Code

Chapter 10
Trust and Regulation as Delegated Understanding

Trust in digital health systems is not an emotion but an operational necessity, permitting action in circumstances where direct verification is impossible. Regulation functions as the societal mechanism through which such verification is delegated: it defines what must be demonstrated for a system to be regarded as trustworthy and distributes responsibility among those who build, evaluate and depend on complex infrastructures. This chapter distinguishes three dimensions of trust—operational, interpretive and epistemic—and argues that interpretive trust, the capacity to understand what was done to data, is now under greatest strain. As data pipelines and AI systems grow in complexity, the documentation they generate exceeds what human-bounded mechanisms of audit and review can absorb. This mismatch is structural rather than operational, arising from the collision between expanding regulatory expectations and the limits of human interpretive capacity. The chapter concludes that sustaining trust at scale will require a shift toward computable forms of assurance, a transition examined in the chapters that follow.

After completing this chapter, readers should be able to:

- Explain why regulation functions as a mechanism for delegating understanding in data-intensive healthcare environments
- Distinguish operational, interpretive and epistemic trust and articulate why interpretive trust is under particular pressure
- Recognise the structural limits of human-bounded documentation and audit at current scales of digital processing

The Concept of Trust in Technical Systems

Trust is often described as a cognitive shortcut (Luhmann 2017). It allows us to act in situations where we cannot personally verify every detail, every mechanism or every risk. Instead of reconstructing an entire causal chain, we accept that a system

M. Bouzinier et al., *Research Data that Can Be Trusted*,
SpringerBriefs in Computer Science, https://doi.org/10.1007/978-3-032-21032-6_10

behaves as expected because the burden of verification has been delegated to someone or something else. In this sense trust is not an emotion but an operational necessity. It reduces uncertainty to a level that enables action.

In healthcare this mechanism is not optional. Clinical practice and health data infrastructures entail layers of abstraction that no individual can oversee in full. A clinician cannot personally validate every diagnostic algorithm or every step in an EHR data pipeline. A researcher cannot inspect each transformation applied to a dataset before it reaches them. A regulator cannot manually recreate the lineage of a dataset used to train an AI model. Yet decisions with clinical, ethical and societal consequences rely on these systems functioning correctly.

Digitalisation amplifies this dynamic. As data flows grow in volume and complexity, the number of intermediaries between cause and effect increases. The more distributed and automated a system becomes, the less visible its inner workings are to those who depend on it. Trust therefore cannot remain a vague social construct. It must be engineered into technical systems through transparency, reproducibility and verifiable adherence to agreed rules.

In this sense trust emerges from two intertwined processes: clarifying what constitutes acceptable practice and creating mechanisms that make conformance observable. These mechanisms rarely arise spontaneously. Societies formalise them in the form of norms, standards and regulatory frameworks that stabilise expectations and manage uncertainty when individual verification is impossible.

Regulation—The Societal Mechanism for Delegating Understanding

When uncertainty exceeds an individual's capacity to assess risk, societies develop mechanisms that stabilise expectations and distribute responsibility. Regulation is one such mechanism. In practice it spans formal law and enforcement, delegated rules, institutional governance and professional consensus standards and guidelines that define acceptable practice and how it should be demonstrated. Among other things, it formalises collective judgement about what is acceptable, what is required and what must never occur when handling sensitive data or designing systems that influence human lives. In this sense regulation does not merely constrain; it structures trust by defining the boundaries within which trust can be rationally placed. This is regulation as delegated understanding, complementing the behavioural delegation that Bar-Gill and Sunstein (Bar-Gill and Sunstein 2015) describe, where boundedly rational individuals cede decision-making authority to government agents. When systems exceed what individuals can verify, regulation defines what evidence must be produced to warrant trust.

This function is especially evident in healthcare, a domain where individuals rely on professionals, institutions and increasingly digital infrastructures to act safely on their behalf. It would be unrealistic for a patient, researcher or policymaker to verify every link in the chain that transforms raw clinical information into evidence or AI-driven insight. Regulation steps in as a proxy for that verification. It articulates minimum safeguards, codifies good practice and establishes obligations for those who build and operate health information systems through statutory requirements where applicable and through standards, accreditation and professional guidance that operationalise those requirements in practice.

Historically these mechanisms first emerged to protect individuals from harm in research and care. In the decades after the Second World War, the Nuremberg Code (1947) and the Declaration of Helsinki (1964, subsequently revised) established explicit ethical boundaries for experimentation on human subjects, encoding the principle that those who cannot protect themselves require institutional safeguards. In subsequent decades these principles were progressively translated into enforceable governance regimes, including national research ethics frameworks and regulatory requirements for clinical research and health information systems.

Later frameworks extended this logic from the protection of the body to the management of information, recognising that misuse of data can be as consequential as misuse of the body. In Europe this included Convention 108, the Data Protection Directive and later the General Data Protection Regulation (GDPR), Clinical Trial Regulation and Medical Devices Regulation. In the United States comparable institutionalisation occurred through instruments such as the Belmont Report, the Common Rule, FDA regulatory requirements and HIPAA.

Regulation thus functions as a contract of expectations between those who create systems, those who evaluate them and those who depend on their outcomes. It specifies the evidence that creators must provide, the criteria that evaluators must apply and the assurances that users can legitimately expect. This contract does not eliminate uncertainty but renders it manageable by defining what must be demonstrated in order for a system to be regarded as trustworthy.

Digitalisation, however, has altered the relationship between regulation and the systems it governs. Modern infrastructures generate large volumes of data and modify that data through layers of automated processing that no individual can reasonably audit in full. AI systems amplify this effect by learning from patterns that are themselves products of complex data preparation pipelines. Regulation demands transparency, traceability and justification, yet the systems to which these demands now apply produce documentation at a scale that exceeds human interpretability.

This creates a structural tension. Regulation needs information about a system in order to assess it and the system generates more information than traditional oversight processes can absorb. As technical complexity rises, regulatory requirements expand. Expanded requirements demand more documentation. More documentation increases the burden on developers, manufacturers and research teams. The authorities responsible for reviewing these materials face the same volume problem from the opposite side. The result is a mismatch between what regulation needs and what manual processes can deliver.

This mismatch does not arise because regulation is ill-conceived. It reflects the limits of mechanisms designed for systems whose behaviours were comprehensible and auditable at human scale. Health data pipelines and AI systems no longer fit that description. Their complexity cannot be managed through procedural checklists, manual audits or interpretive reviews alone. Regulation continues to function as a societal instrument for delegating understanding and stabilising trust, but it increasingly lacks the means to operationalise that function. Without new tools and methods, compliance and oversight are in danger of becoming symbolic rather than substantive.

The Dual Function of Regulation in Data-Intensive Systems

Regulation serves two complementary functions in domains where risks cannot be evaluated by individuals alone. It has a protective function, grounded in the obligation to prevent harm, and an enabling function, aimed at creating the conditions under which complex systems can operate reliably at scale. Both aspects are present in healthcare, and both gain importance as systems become more data-intensive and more dependent on automated processes.

The protective function is the most familiar. It encompasses requirements intended to safeguard individuals and to prevent foreseeable forms of harm, including:

- safety,
- fairness,
- non-maleficence,
- privacy.

These obligations define boundaries for the collection, transformation, sharing and secondary use of health data. They protect individuals from disproportionate risks and ensure that emerging technologies do not amplify existing inequities or introduce new forms of harm. In practice this translates into procedural safeguards, documentation duties and constraints on permissible data uses, all aimed at reducing uncertainty for those who cannot evaluate risks directly.

But we should never forget that the enabling function is equally fundamental. Regulation provides shared structures that allow different actors, organisations and technical systems to interact without continuous renegotiation of rules. Elements of this enabling role include:

- standardisation,
- interoperability,
- reproducibility.

These requirements stabilise a domain where many parties contribute partial components of larger processes. They reduce friction, encourage comparability and support the formation of ecosystems in which data and models can circulate with predictable properties. Without them, data-intensive environments would fragment into incompatible practices that undermine their intended purposes.

The rise of data-intensive systems has strengthened both functions. As health data pipelines grow in complexity and scale, and as AI systems rely on increasingly elaborate transformations, the protective obligations expand accordingly. At the same time, the need for shared standards, precise documentation and reproducible processes becomes more urgent. Regulation therefore acts not only as a boundary but as an infrastructure that supports coordinated activity in environments where manual verification is no longer feasible.

These two functions generate substantial amounts of required information. Each protective requirement creates documentation that must be produced and reviewed. Each enabling requirement introduces expectations for standardisation and formalisation. In data-intensive settings the combined effect is an accelerating volume of regulatory artefacts—what we suggest calling a ***volume crisis***—amplifying the structural mismatch described in the preceding section. Before examining how this mismatch might be addressed, it is necessary to distinguish more precisely what is meant by trust in digital health systems, since different dimensions of trust face different pressures and require different interventions.

The Three Dimensions of Trust in Digital Health

Trust in digital health systems has traditionally been discussed along two axes: the security of the environment in which data are handled and the reliability of the results produced. These two dimensions remain central, yet they no longer capture the full landscape. As data pipelines become more automated and as regulatory expectations expand, a third dimension becomes essential: the ability to understand and verify the processes through which results are generated. We distinguish the three dimensions of trust to clarify the pressures facing contemporary systems and the types of interventions required to sustain it.

Operational trust concerns the secure and predictable functioning of the technical infrastructure. It relates to how data are stored, how access is controlled and how misuse can be prevented or detected. Elements include encryption, access management, audit logging and resilience of the underlying environment. These measures ensure that data remains protected from unauthorised access and that systems behave reliably at an infrastructural level. The engineering disciplines that support operational trust are mature and grounded in well established practices.

Interpretive trust concerns the transparency of data processes. It relates to the ability to trace and understand what happens to data as it moves through a pipeline: which transformations were applied, which assumptions shaped these transformations and how intermediate steps contribute to the final output. Interpretive trust does not require access to raw data but requires a verifiable account of the logic applied to it. This includes explicit transformation rules, structured documentation and machine-readable lineage that allow independent reproduction or audit. As pipelines grow in complexity, manual inspection and informal documentation are no longer sufficient.

Provenance and clear semantics become necessary to articulate how results were produced.

Epistemic trust concerns acceptance of the results themselves. The term has a longer history in social epistemology, where it typically refers to reliance on others for knowledge one cannot independently verify (Hardwig 1991). We use it in a narrower sense: trust that analytical outputs such as predictions, model results and derived statistics are valid for their intended purpose. Epistemic trust depends on the other two dimensions. A secure system cannot compensate for opaque processing logic, and transparent processing cannot substitute for empirical validation of the result.

Example:

A machine learning pipeline may be operationally trustworthy: containerised, versioned and executed in a controlled environment. Yet interpretive trust fails if key preprocessing steps such as collapsing age bands, removing rare events or imputing missing values are implemented without formal documentation. When the resulting model behaves differently across subgroups, neither developers nor reviewers can explain why. Epistemic trust becomes uncertain because the logic that shaped the data remains opaque.

While these dimensions address different concerns, they are tightly connected. Operational trust provides the conditions under which data can be handled safely. Interpretive trust provides the transparency needed to understand how outputs were produced. Epistemic trust provides confidence that these outputs can be relied upon. As the scale and complexity of digital health systems increase, pressures concentrate on the interpretive layer, where the transparency of data processes becomes essential for sustaining trust.

The Limit of Scale for Human-Bounded Trust Mechanisms

Regulation provides a formal structure for trust, yet the mechanisms through which this structure is operationalised remain predominantly human. Documentation is written by people, audits are performed by people and the interpretation of compliance depends on human judgement. These mechanisms were adequate when systems were simpler, data volumes were moderate and the behaviour of technological artefacts could be inspected and understood directly.

Data-intensive systems have altered these conditions. Modern health data pipelines involve many layers of transformation, each of which may introduce assumptions, intermediate states or implicit decisions that are difficult to describe concisely. AI systems compound this by producing stochastic outputs learned from statistical patterns rather than explicit, interpretable rules. The documentation required to understand and evaluate such systems expands proportionally to their complexity. Human-bounded mechanisms struggle with this expansion because the amount of information to be produced and interpreted grows faster than our capacity to process it.

Manual documentation becomes inconsistent or incomplete, not because individuals are careless but because the task exceeds what can reasonably be maintained. Manual audits risk becoming symbolic when the volume of artefacts outpaces what can be reviewed in depth. Human interpretation becomes a bottleneck when each assessment requires reconstructing chains of transformations that are opaque or only partially recorded. The cumulative effect is a procedural saturation: the formal frameworks remain intact, but the means of fulfilling them no longer keep pace with the systems they are meant to govern.

This is a structural problem rather than an operational one. It stems from the mismatch between human interpretive capacity and the complexity of modern data processing. The interpretive dimension of trust, which depends on understanding how data were shaped, is the most vulnerable. Without new methods to formalise and render these processes computable, trust cannot be sustained in a reliable or scalable way.

The shift from human-bounded to computable trust does not replace human judgement but supports it. It provides a foundation on which evaluators can rely without reconstructing the full internal logic of a system. The next chapter examines how this shift becomes unavoidable once regulatory expectations and technical complexity converge to produce a volume crisis.

References

Bar-Gill, O., & Sunstein, C. R. (2015). Regulation as Delegation. *Journal of Legal Analysis*, *7*(1), 1–36. https://doi.org/10.1093/jla/lav005.

Hardwig, J. (1991). The Role of Trust in Knowledge. *The Journal of Philosophy*, *88*(12), 693–708. https://doi.org/10.2307/2027007.

Luhmann, N. (2017). *Trust and Power*. Polity Press.

Chapter 11
The Burden Spiral: When Technology Exceeds Human Oversight

This chapter describes how digital health systems moved from contained, institution-centric setups to distributed pipelines that span organisations, jurisdictions, and modalities. As context becomes dispersed, oversight increasingly operates at a distance, so it shifts from rule-following to evidence-based assessment of concrete data processes. Governance diversifies in parallel, not only through laws and policy, but also through standards, professional guidance, accreditation and procurement requirements that become quasi-mandatory in practice. The result is a "burden spiral" or volume crisis: more documentation is requested and produced, yet human-bounded review cannot absorb it, so additional evidence does not yield proportional understanding and trust deteriorates. The chapter argues that this is a structural limit of oversight models that rely on documents written for human interpretation, and it sets up the need for a different evidentiary substrate in the next chapter.

After completing this chapter, readers should be able to:

- Explain why modern health data systems create interpretive distance through distributed pipelines, federated analytics, and multimodal data
- Describe how governance diversification, including standards and professional guidance, increases evidentiary demands while review capacity remains bounded
- Define the burden spiral as a structural volume crisis and explain why incremental documentation cannot resolve it

The Changing Structure of Digital Complexity

Contemporary health data systems are widely acknowledged to be complex, and this complexity has grown steadily over the past two decades. As digitalisation advanced in the early 2000s, hospitals and research institutions expanded their electronic record systems, introduced large-scale registries and began to link administrative and clinical data for analytical purposes. By the 2010s, applications of big data, data lakes

M. Bouzinier et al., *Research Data that Can Be Trusted*,
SpringerBriefs in Computer Science, https://doi.org/10.1007/978-3-032-21032-6_11

and distributed analytical architectures had become common across the health sector. These developments increased the amount of information available and broadened the range of technologies used to process it, yet we can see them as gradual improvement rather than transformational. Institutions continued to operate within defined perimeters, and while technical challenges accumulated, the context in which data were produced and interpreted remained accessible to those responsible for their use within the predefined boundaries.

The past decade has altered these conditions. Pressures for cross-institutional collaboration have intensified, driven in part by global health emergencies (World Health Organization 2023) that demonstrated the limitations of isolated information systems and the need for rapid, coordinated access to data. Simultaneously, concerns about privacy, sovereignty and strategic dependency have led to stronger regional and national controls over data flows. These opposing forces reshape digital infrastructures in parallel: they encourage the integration of diverse datasets across organisations and sectors, yet they also impose governance requirements that restrict centralisation and mandate that data remain within specific legal or operational boundaries. Analytical work increasingly depends on interacting with data that cannot be freely moved, fully inspected or standardised in a single location.

Within this environment, national research data infrastructures have emerged to bridge fragmented landscapes. Initiatives like Health Data Research in the United Kingdom, Health-RI in the Netherlands (*Health-RI | Health-RI* n.d.) or All-of-Us in the United States (The All of Us Research Program Investigators 2019) were created to bridge datasets dispersed across health systems, research centres and public bodies, providing common governance structures for analytical use. They acknowledge that no single organisation holds either the volume or diversity of data needed for contemporary research and that meaningful analysis requires coordination across institutional and jurisdictional lines. Yet these infrastructures do not eliminate local variation. They operate on top of heterogeneous operational practices, data qualities and historical conventions that persist within their contributing institutions.

At the technical level, analytical processes have shifted from monolithic systems to distributed pipelines. Instead of a contained sequence of operations, data now flow through chains that handle extraction, linkage, harmonisation, feature construction, model training and evaluation across multiple environments. Multimodal architectures combine structured records with images, free-text documents and sensor streams. Machine-learned systems apply long sequences of automated transformations whose intermediate states are not routinely observed. The behaviour of such systems emerges from interactions between components that evolve independently, and understanding it requires insight into processes that may be situated far upstream from the point where results are consumed (McMurry et al. 2007).

Federated analytical models add another layer of structural change. In response to privacy and sovereignty requirements, many organisations now operate under constraints that prevent data from leaving their institutional or national boundaries. Analytical methods that distribute computation across sites, or that train models locally while aggregating only statistical updates, address these constraints (Casaletto et al. 2023). However, they also mean that results depend on assumptions and practices embedded in environments that participants cannot fully observe. The apparent unity of a shared model thus conceals a heterogeneous landscape of local preprocessing routines, coding conventions and data qualities that influence outcomes without being explicitly visible.

These developments have been accompanied by a diversification of governance. International organisations articulate principles for responsible data use, regional authorities introduce sector-specific obligations and national institutions develop their own models for access, retention and accountability. Evaluation of the growing number of data governance frameworks (Hassani et al. 2025) identifies a rapid proliferation of initiatives across scientific and public domains, reflecting a broad recognition that coordination is necessary in distributed data environments. Yet each framework embodies assumptions about risk, purpose and acceptable practice that may differ across jurisdictions and sectors. The result is not a unified governance regime but an overlapping set of expectations that shape how data can be processed and shared.

Taken together, these trends have produced a form of complexity that cannot be understood solely in terms of the sophistication of individual technologies. The defining characteristic is the distribution of context across many systems and institutions. Processes that span organisational boundaries carry assumptions that are invisible to downstream actors. Harmonisation routines, cohort definitions and preprocessing decisions made upstream propagate through analytical chains without being explicitly communicated. As pipelines and governance regimes evolve independently, the interpretive distance between data producers, data processors and data consumers increases. Those who rely on analytical outputs must trust results whose provenance is not readily accessible, not because systems fail but because the relations that shape their behaviour are not captured in forms that can be easily interpreted.

This structural transformation alters the basis on which trust can be sustained. It is no longer sufficient to assume that the behaviour of a system can be understood by examining its components or reviewing human-written documentation. Understanding modern digital ecosystems requires a means of recovering how data have been shaped as they traverse dispersed technical and institutional environments. Without such means the informational foundation of trust becomes fragile, as the processes that generate results become increasingly opaque to those who depend on them.

Oversight Under Governance Diversity

As digital infrastructures extend across institutions and jurisdictions, oversight must operate at a distance from the processes it is meant to evaluate. In more contained settings, accountability could rely on organisational proximity: those responsible for review knew the systems, the actors and the local conventions that shaped data processing. Diversified ecosystems break this link. Common in clinical research, data collected in one context, e.g., at the point of care, may have been extracted, linked and transformed for secondary use by researchers, clinical investigators or auditors. The bodies charged with granting approvals or assessing conformity cannot rely on implicit knowledge of how systems behave and must therefore request more explicit evidence before accepting that risks are controlled and claims about performance are justified.

This shift gradually transforms oversight from a rule-following to evidence assessment. Formal requirements still take the form of obligations and prohibitions, but their practical implementation depends increasingly on showing how data are handled in concrete systems (Burns et al. 2022). Descriptions of sources, inclusion criteria, preprocessing steps, validation procedures and monitoring arrangements become central, not incidental, to regulatory interaction. Each change in a pipeline, model or data source potentially alters the basis on which earlier approvals were granted and with it the need to update the evidentiary record. Documentation grows because systems evolve and because oversight now depends on the ability to reconstruct, at least in principle, the path from raw data to result (Carl and Hochmann 2024).

At the same time, governance itself is no longer singular. Organisations are subject to layers of expectations arising from data protection law, sector-specific regulation, research ethics, contractual obligations and the governance rules of shared infrastructures. These frameworks are not identical in their concepts or thresholds, yet they all rely on the availability of information about how data are collected, transformed and used. Meeting their combined demands requires organisations to generate and maintain a growing body of technical and procedural artefacts: protocols, risk assessments, data flow descriptions, validation reports and change histories. Oversight bodies, in turn, must interpret this material in light of the frameworks they apply, often without direct access to the systems that produced it.

The means of evaluation, however, remain predominantly human. Whether located in regulatory authorities, data access committees or institutional review boards, oversight depends on experts reading documents, examining selected technical artefacts and forming judgements about adequacy and residual risk. Their capacity is finite. The more diversified the ecosystem and the more frequently systems change, the greater the volume and granularity of information that would need to be considered to sustain interpretive trust. At a certain point, additional documentation no longer translates into proportional understanding. Reviewers cannot reconstruct complex chains of transformation from narrative descriptions and scattered machine-generated outputs within the time and cognitive limits available to them.

Oversight under conditions of heterogeneity therefore faces a structural limit. It must request more evidence because context is no longer shared, yet it can only process a fraction of what it receives. The result is a growing gap between the descriptive prerequisites of trust and the human mechanisms available to assess them. This gap is not a temporary resourcing issue but a consequence of how modern data ecosystems are organised, and it marks the point at which human-bounded review reaches its natural limits.

Standards and Professional Guidance as a Quasi-regulatory Layer

Governance pressure does not come only from statutes and formal oversight bodies. A large share comes from professional standards, technical specifications, accreditation criteria and clinical guidance that translate abstract duties into concrete expectations about how data and pipelines should be built, validated and monitored. In clinical genomics, for example, the credibility of an interpretation workflow is judged not only against privacy or data protection law but also against professional guidance such as American College of Medical Genetics and Genomics (ACMG) (Richards et al. 2015) classification criteria, laboratory accreditation regimes such as College of American Pathologists—a voluntary accreditation that meets U.S. federal law of Clinical Laboratory Improvement Amendments (*Clinical Laboratory Improvement Amendments of* 1988). Similar dynamics apply across imaging, pathology, device software and clinical decision support.

This layer becomes quasi-regulatory because it shapes what is practically acceptable, even when it is not formally mandatory. There are several mechanisms. *First*, regulators increasingly reference standards as a pathway to conformity. When a legal regime is written in technology-neutral language, it often delegates operational detail to standards, profiles and "state of the art" expectations. *Second*, accreditation and certification bodies operationalise requirements through checklists, controls and evidence templates, turning broad obligations into a recurring audit workload. *Third*, procurement and contracting embed standards as conditions of participation: compliance becomes a precondition for market access, reimbursement, or partnership, not just a legal risk (Australian Government 2024). *Fourth*, professional and clinical communities enforce norms through peer review, reputational risk and liability expectations. In practice, teams that deviate from widely accepted guidance must carry an evidentiary burden to justify why.

The consequence is that governance heterogeneity is not only law-to-law or regulator-to-regulator. It is also law-to-standard, standard-to-standard and guideline-to-guideline. Technical standards from Standards Development Organizations (SDO) such as ISO, IEC, HL7, IHE, IEEE and domain-specific profiles frequently intersect with organisational policies, research ethics requirements and platform rules inside shared infrastructures. They are updated on their own cycles, use their own terminology and often assume different "units of evidence" than legal texts. A system may be expected to produce one package of evidence for regulatory conformity, another for accreditation, another for internal quality management and another for procurement assurance, all describing overlapping realities in different formats.

This is where a common misconception needs to be unpacked: standards can reduce ambiguity, but they do not automatically reduce workload. They compress interpretation in one place, but they multiply interfaces elsewhere. Each additional standard introduces mapping work, version tracking, profile selection and documentation obligations. Interoperability standards often require local implementation choices that must be recorded and defended. Security and privacy standards introduce control catalogs and monitoring expectations. Clinical guidance introduces domain-specific validation and change-control expectations. The organisation then carries not only the operational work, but also the work of demonstrating alignment across these layers.

The update dynamic matters as much as the content. Standards evolve, profiles fork and best practice shifts. A pipeline that was "aligned" last year may no longer be aligned today, even if its code did not change, because the reference baseline moved. In distributed ecosystems, different actors may operate on different versions of the "same" standard, or interpret the same profile differently. The evidentiary record must therefore track not only what the system does, but which standard version, which profile, which interpretation and which exceptions were used and why.

In short, professional standards and guidance amplify the documentation economy that the previous section describes. They do not replace statutory governance, they thicken it. Oversight asks for evidence that a system is safe and trustworthy and the fastest way to answer is to point to standards alignment, yet alignment itself expands the volume of artefacts that must be produced, updated and interpreted. The result is more documentation, more crosswalks and more opportunities for drift between what is implemented and what is claimed.

The Burden Spiral as a Structural Outcome

The dynamics described in the preceding sections can be framed more precisely as a volume crisis. Modern digital ecosystems generate evidentiary material at a rate and granularity that exceed what human-bounded oversight can absorb. Each additional data source, transformation step or model variant introduces new potential points of failure and new justifications that, in principle, ought to be documented if trust is to be maintained. At the same time, each new governance layer or regulatory framework extends the range of questions that documentation is expected to answer. The quantity of information that would be needed to support a fully informed judgement grows faster than the capacity of any institution to process it.

Evidence of this imbalance is already visible. The OECD policy observatory (Organisation for Economic Co-operation and Development (OECD) 2024) tracks over seven hundred AI-related initiatives across more than eighty jurisdictions, reflecting the scale of governance proliferation. Industry bodies have documented the cumulative administrative burden of overlapping medical devices and diagnostic regulations (Europe 2025). Professional associations responsible for conformity assessment have warned that capacity constraints risk undermining the implementation of new frameworks such as the EU AI Act (Denoon and King n.d.). These are not projections of a future difficulty but descriptions of conditions already in effect. The volume crisis is not approaching; it has arrived.

This crisis has three interrelated dimensions. The first is scale: the absolute volume of artefacts produced by routine operation of data pipelines and analytical systems rises as infrastructures become more interconnected and automation increases. The second is granularity: evidentiary expectations move from high-level descriptions towards fine-grained accounts of data provenance, model behaviour and contextual performance, multiplying the number of details that matter. The third is tempo: systems and their environments change more frequently than oversight cycles, so that by the time documentation has been reviewed, the underlying configurations may already have shifted. Together these dimensions create a widening gap between what would be required for genuine interpretive trust and what can be examined through manual review.

The gap has material consequences for both sides of the regulatory relationship. On the side of those who build and operate systems, preparing submissions that satisfy proliferating evidentiary expectations consumes increasing amounts of time and resources. Teams that might otherwise focus on improving data quality, refining models or validating results must devote substantial effort to assembling, updating and aligning documentation with evolving requirements. For smaller organisations this effort can become a decisive barrier to innovation. On the side of those who evaluate systems, limited capacity leads to queues, backlogs and pressure to prioritise certain applications over others. Even when evaluators work at the limits of their capacity, they cannot review all submissions in the depth that the formal requirements imply.

When oversight bodies fall behind, they request clearer or more standardised submissions to reduce interpretive effort. Applicants respond by investing in documentation that conforms to expected templates, diverting resources from substantive improvement. As submissions become more uniform, reviewers lose the contextual signals that once helped distinguish genuinely robust systems from well-packaged weak ones and compensate by requesting additional detail. Each adaptation intended to manage the burden generates conditions that intensify it. Organisations learn to produce artefacts that satisfy formal expectations without necessarily advancing understanding. Evaluators, confronted with more material than they can interpret, rely on heuristics: conformity to established patterns, reputation of applicants, familiarity with particular technologies. Decisions continue to be taken, but they rest on partial readings of the evidentiary record. The formal structure of trust remains intact while its informational foundation erodes. The dynamic is self-reinforcing, manifesting in the spiral of burden.

The volume crisis therefore marks more than an administrative overload. It signals a structural limit of a governance model in which trust is mediated through documents intended for human interpretation. As long as the informational preconditions of trust expand along the trajectories described and as long as evaluation remains constrained by human cognitive and organisational capacities, the burden spiral cannot be resolved by incremental adjustments (Cimolino et al. 2023). Additional requirements, more detailed guidance or greater diligence may delay its effects, but they do not change the underlying imbalance. The consequence is a gradual erosion of interpretive trust in the systems being assessed and, in parallel, a strain on institutional trust in the bodies responsible for their oversight.

Trust, however, does not disappear simply because existing mechanisms for sustaining it reach their limits. The structural imbalance described in this chapter forces a different question: if documentation written for human interpretation can no longer carry the evidentiary weight placed upon it, what other forms of representation could support interpretive trust under conditions of scale and diversification. Addressing the volume crisis then becomes less a matter of adding further layers of control and more a matter of reconfiguring the substrate on which evidence about data and systems is recorded. The next chapter examines provenance in this light, not as a marginal technical detail, but as the infrastructural element that determines whether complex data processes can be rendered interpretable in a way that is compatible with the constraints of contemporary oversight.

References

Australian Government. (2024). *Policy for the responsible use of AI in government—Version 2.0.* Digital Transformation Agency. https://architecture.digital.gov.au/policy/responsible-use-of-ai-in-government

Burns, L., Roux, N. L., Kalesnik-Orszulak, R., Christian, J., Hukkelhoven, M., Rockhold, F., & O'Donnell, J. (2022). Real-World Evidence for Regulatory Decision-Making: Guidance From Around the World. *Clinical Therapeutics, 44*(3), 420–437. https://doi.org/10.1016/j.clinthera.2022.01.012.

Carl, A.-K., & Hochmann, D. (2024). Impact of the new European medical device regulation: A two-year comparison. *Biomedical Engineering/Biomedizinische Technik, 69*(3), 317–326. https://doi.org/10.1515/bmt-2023-0325.

Casaletto, J., Bernier, A., McDougall, R., & Cline, M. S. (2023). Federated Analysis for Privacy-Preserving Data Sharing: A Technical and Legal Primer. *Annual Review of Genomics and Human Genetics, 24*(Volume 24, 2023), 347–368. https://doi.org/10.1146/annurev-genom-110122-084756.

Cimolino, G., Chen, R. (Xinyu), Gutwin, C., & Graham, T. C. N. (2023). Automation Confusion: A Grounded Theory of Non-Gamers' Confusion in Partially Automated Action Games. *Proceedings of the 2023 CHI Conference on Human Factors in Computing Systems.* https://doi.org/10.1145/3544548.3581116.

Clinical Laboratory Improvement Amendments of 1988. (1988). https://www.govinfo.gov/content/pkg/USCODE-2011-title42/pdf/USCODE-2011-title42-chap6A-subchapII-partF-subpart2-sec263a.pdf

Denoon, A., & King, M. (n.d.). EU AI Act: Will regulation drive innovation away from Europe? *European Pharmaceutical Review.* Retrieved December 29, 2025, from https://www.europeanpharmaceuticalreview.com/article/238250/the-eu-ai-act-will-regulation-drive-life-science-innovation-away-from-europe/

Europe, M. (2025). *Report on Administrative Burden under IVDR and MDR.* MedTech Europe. https://www.medtecheurope.org/resource-library/medtech-europes-report-on-administrative-burden-under-ivdr-and-mdr/

Hassani, H., Huang, X., & MacFeely, S. (2025). Mapping the evolution of data governance scientific research. *Data & Policy, 7*, e51. https://doi.org/10.1017/dap.2025.10014.

Health-RI | Health-RI. (n.d.). Retrieved December 29, 2025, from https://www.health-ri.nl/en/health-ri

McMurry, A. J., Gilbert, C. A., Reis, B. Y., Chueh, H. C., Kohane, I. S., & Mandl, K. D. (2007). A Self-scaling, Distributed Information Architecture for Public Health, Research, and Clinical Care. *Journal of the American Medical Informatics Association, 14*(4), 527–533. https://doi.org/10.1197/jamia.M2371.

Organisation for Economic Co-operation and Development (OECD). (2024). *Policies, data and analysis for trustworthy artificial intelligence.* https://oecd.ai/en/

Richards, S., Aziz, N., Bale, S., Bick, D., Das, S., Gastier-Foster, J., Grody, W. W., Hegde, M., Lyon, E., Spector, E., Voelkerding, K., & Rehm, H. L. (2015). Standards and guidelines for the interpretation of sequence variants: A joint consensus recommendation of the American College of Medical Genetics and Genomics and the Association for Molecular Pathology. *Genetics in Medicine, 17*(5), 405–423. https://doi.org/10.1038/gim.2015.30.

The All of Us Research Program Investigators. (2019). The "All of Us" Research Program. *New England Journal of Medicine, 381*(7), 668–676. https://doi.org/10.1056/NEJMsr1809937.

World Health Organization. (2023). *Global Research and Innovation for Health Emergencies: Building the World's Resilience Against Future Outbreaks and Pandemics* [WHO Report]. World Health Organization. https://cdn.who.int/media/docs/default-source/documents/r-d-blueprint-meetings/global-research-and-innovation-for-health-emergencies_report-2023.pdf

Chapter 12
The Provenance Imperative

Introduction

This chapter argues that the bottleneck is not only the volume of documentation, but the way information about data processes is represented. Current practice concentrates on environments, actors and dataset-level lineage, while leaving transformation logic dispersed across code, notebooks and narrative artefacts. Meanwhile, regulatory and governance frameworks in Europe and beyond increasingly assume that process-level knowledge exists and can be supplied on demand, without specifying how it should be captured or expressed. We interpret this as an implicit requirement for transformation-level provenance and introduce actionable provenance: structured records of data transformations that are automatically captured, portable and machine-interpretable.

After completing this chapter, readers should be able to:

- Explain why interpretive trust breaks down as a representational problem, not merely an overload of documentation
- Distinguish dataset-level lineage and conventional provenance artefacts from transformation-level, semantic provenance and explain the practical limits of current approaches
- Define actionable provenance and connect its core properties to the kinds of evidence implicitly demanded by modern health data and AI governance

From Volume Crisis to a Problem of Representation

The volume crisis described in the previous chapter is often portrayed as a simple imbalance between the amount of information that systems produce and the capacity of institutions to review it. This description is incomplete. The growth in documentation and technical artefacts is not accidental; it arises from legitimate expectations

M. Bouzinier et al., *Research Data that Can Be Trusted*,
SpringerBriefs in Computer Science, https://doi.org/10.1007/978-3-032-21032-6_12

that systems handling health data should be safe, ethically defensible, resistant to bias, sensitive to diversity and protective of the individuals whose data they use. To claim that these expectations are met, actors must provide some account of how datasets were assembled, how variables were constructed and how models were trained and evaluated. Regulatory instruments and governance frameworks increasingly reflect this logic, even when they do not specify precisely what such an account should contain. As a result, organisations generate protocols, data flow diagrams, risk assessments and descriptive reports that attempt to demonstrate that their pipelines embody the safeguards they claim. The volume crisis is therefore rooted in an obligation to show that systems deserve trust, not in a taste for bureaucracy.

Yet the form in which this information is produced remains poorly aligned with the needs it is supposed to serve. As established in the previous chapter, documentation is largely written for human readers and refers to code, scripts and configuration artefacts that themselves are difficult to interpret or reproduce outside the original context. Even when code repositories are complete and versioned, they rarely provide a direct answer to questions about how a particular dataset was shaped, which assumptions governed inclusion and exclusion, or which parameter choices materially affected the representation of subgroups. Conversely, narrative documentation often abstracts away from implementation details in order to remain readable, leaving out precisely the elements that would be necessary to assess the impact of transformations on bias, diversity or privacy. The result is an accumulation of materials that point to each other without forming a coherent picture of what has been done to the data.

This misalignment becomes more acute as systems evolve rapidly. Pipelines and models are revised to accommodate new data sources, updated algorithms or corrected errors. Each change introduces further details that ought to be reflected in the accompanying documentation if earlier claims about safety, fairness or robustness are to remain valid. In practice, the pace of modification exceeds what can be captured consistently in human-authored texts. References to scripts and notebooks become outdated, links to repositories lose synchrony with deployed versions and the informal knowledge held by teams drifts away from what is recorded. The frequency of change, the granularity of decisions embedded in code and configuration and the distribution of responsibilities across institutions together make it increasingly unlikely that any single actor could reconstruct, from available artefacts, a reliable account of how a given result was produced.

The bottleneck in interpretive trust is therefore not only quantitative but representational (Mitchell et al. 2019). It is not simply that there is too much information, but that the information is structured in ways that fragment the sequence of decisions and transformations into pieces that cannot be easily recombined. Narrative descriptions and free-form technical reports describe aspects of processes without providing a consistent, reusable way of expressing how they compose into complete pipelines. Code and scripts encode exact behaviour but in a form that is opaque to most reviewers and brittle across platforms. Between these two extremes, a stable layer is missing that captures, in a systematic manner, what was actually done to data in terms that can be related to the expectations embodied in regulatory and ethical frameworks. Provenance, understood as a structured account of the transformations applied to data and the conditions under which they were applied, points to how such a layer could be constructed.

Current Provenance Practice

Provenance is not a new concern in health and research data. Many infrastructures already record aspects of how data are handled and make these records available for audit and governance. Trusted research environments maintain access logs that show which users connected to which datasets under which approvals. Data warehouses and analytical platforms often record dataset-level lineage, indicating which input tables were combined to produce a given output and, in some cases, linking to code repositories where transformation scripts are stored. Generic provenance models such as the World Wide Web Consortium's PROV family of specifications for modelling provenance metadata represent relations between entities, activities and agents in a uniform graph, providing a common language for describing which processes produced which artefacts. Domain-specific initiatives in clinical data warehouses and quality management, including provenance frameworks inspired by projects such as Standardised Architecture for Trusted Research Environments (SATRE) (Cole et al. 2023), document extraction, transformation and loading steps at the level of tables or data flows, often with the aim of improving traceability and data quality. The FAIR Data Principles introduced by Mark D. Wilkinson et al. in 2016 (Wilkinson et al. 2016) to improve on findability, accessibility, interoperability and reusability (FAIR) of data for scientific research, advocate for metadata profiles extended with information about origin, formats, licensing and governance arrangements, sometimes including high-level accounts of processing steps.

These approaches answer several important questions. They make it possible to reconstruct, at least in outline, where a dataset came from and which systems contributed to its creation. They allow institutions to demonstrate that access to sensitive data occurred within approved projects and under defined conditions. They help identify which versions of a script or workflow were used to produce a result and which environment hosted the execution. They support internal quality initiatives by showing which pipelines populate which data marts and how updates propagate through a warehouse. They also provide a means to show that data have been handled within specified governance frameworks, for example by documenting that they were processed inside a particular secure infrastructure or under a specific contractual regime. In this sense, existing provenance practice supports operational accountability, platform management and legal defensibility: it documents who did what, where and when.

However, these forms of provenance are less suited to answering questions about what was actually done to the data in a way that affects interpretive trust. They rarely capture the detailed semantics of transformations, such as how variables were recoded, which imputation methods were applied to which fields, how rare categories were handled or which aggregation rules were used to construct composite indicators. Cohort definitions are often described in free text or encoded in queries that are not preserved in an interpretable form. Feature engineering steps that derive new variables from raw measures, normalise distributions or apply domain-specific thresholds are embedded in code rather than surfaced as structured, inspectable decisions. Parameter choices that materially influence analytic validity or bias typically remain implicit in scripts or configuration files, if they are recorded at all. Even where W3C PROV-style graphs or warehouse provenance frameworks are used, they tend to describe the existence of a transformation activity and its inputs and outputs, not the internal logic by which values were reshaped.

Typical limitations follow from these omissions. Many provenance records are constructed retrospectively and selectively, assembled once a project is underway or approaching completion. They rely on manual effort and are therefore vulnerable to gaps, simplifications and inconsistencies. Others are tightly coupled to specific tools or platforms, making it difficult to transfer their meaning when data move between systems. Most are designed with human readers in mind: they take the form of logs, diagrams or narrative descriptions that can be inspected in isolation, but are not easily combined or analysed systematically across many pipelines and projects. As a result, they provide assurance that certain procedural requirements were followed and that data were handled within appropriate environments, yet they offer only limited insight into the chains of transformation that shaped the content of datasets and model inputs.

By outlining these observations, the last thing we want to do is to diminish the value of existing provenance mechanisms for the purposes they were designed to serve. These mechanisms remain essential for demonstrating compliance with access controls, documenting the use of sensitive data, managing complex data warehouses and satisfying requirements related to security and governance. But their limitations become apparent when provenance is expected to carry a different burden, namely to support interpretive trust in settings where data are repeatedly reshaped through long, automated pipelines and where regulatory expectations extend into the details of data preparation. In such settings, knowing who accessed which dataset, which script ran where and which table fed which data mart is not sufficient to form a reasoned judgement about how results were produced. Without a reliable, computable account of the transformations applied to data, provenance cannot fully address the challenges that arise when scale and diversification render human-bounded interpretation of code and documentation impractical.

Regulatory and Governance Signals of the Provenance Imperative

From Environments to Processes

Regulatory frameworks in health and AI were originally constructed around environments and actors. They sought to ensure that data were stored in secure systems, accessed only for approved purposes, governed by appropriate consent or contractual arrangements and handled by identifiable organisations under clear responsibility. These elements remain present, yet recent instruments increasingly direct their attention to the internal processes that shape data and models. Requirements now address how training, validation and test datasets are assembled and governed, how preprocessing is carried out, how model performance is monitored under real-world conditions and how changes in data or algorithms are managed over time. The object of oversight thus shifts from the environment around a system to the sequences of transformations within it.

European AI Regulation

European instruments make the shift from environments to processes unusually explicit and, in doing so, expose the gap between legal expectations and the structures presently available in most data pipelines. For high-risk systems of which many healthcare applications are (AI Act, Article 6), the AI Act requires that training, validation and testing datasets be subject to data governance and management practices "appropriate for the intended purpose" and specifies that these practices must address design choices, data collection processes, the origin and context of data, preparation steps and potential biases, including their detection and mitigation (AI Act, Article 10). It couples these requirements with a general obligation to maintain a risk management system across the lifecycle of a system and to draw on logs and performance records when re-evaluating risks.

A distinctive feature of European governance is its reliance on standards as an operational bridge between law and engineering practice. The AI Act is written in technology-neutral terms, but the compliance pathway is expected to run through harmonised standards, common specifications and conformity assessment practice. The AI Act's harmonization standards were commissioned to CEN and CENELEC (European standardization organizations) to provide technical specifications for compliance, especially for high-risk AI systems (AI Act, Article 40). Once harmonised standards are referenced in the Official Journal, their use can provide a presumption of conformity with relevant legal requirements. In practice, this turns standards into a substrate of oversight: voluntary in principle, but frequently the default way to evidence data governance, risk management, documentation and monitoring and a layer that evolves on its own update cycle (Kilian et al. 2025).

Technical documentation obligations go further by demanding that providers be able to describe, in a structured way, the datasets used for training, validation and testing, their provenance, the criteria for inclusion and exclusion and the preprocessing, cleaning and transformation steps applied to them (AI Act, Article 11 and Annex IV). Guidance emerging around these provisions, including templates for technical documentation developed by conformity assessment bodies, illustrates the level of detail expected: descriptions of how missing data were handled, how outliers were treated, how variables were normalised or encoded, which external data sources were linked and how frequently data are updated. Taken at face value, this implies that providers should be able to reconstruct the internal logic of their data preparation pipelines, not merely list the files and systems involved.

European Regulation of Health Data

The European Health Data Space (EHDS) Regulation moves in a parallel direction from the perspective of secondary use. It establishes a framework under which health data access bodies can grant permits for the reuse of electronic health data for research, innovation and policy, subject to conditions on data quality, interoperability and privacy (EHDS Regulation, Chap. IV, especially Article 68). The regulation mandates, among other elements, labelling of health datasets to indicate their quality and suitability for specific secondary uses (EHDS Regulation, Article 78). Work under the first and second Joint Action Towards the European Health Data Space (TEHDAS) and adjacent EU-funded projects such as QUANTUM—an EU-funded project that aims to create a common label system for Europe—interprets this labelling requirement as encompassing not only source characteristics but also information about how data have been curated, transformed and harmonised for cross-border use. The emerging data quality frameworks link fitness-for-purpose directly to transparency about the manipulations that produce analytical datasets from source records.

The legal pattern is similar to the AI Act. The regulation sets out rights and responsibilities, but the day-to-day mechanics of discoverability and reuse depend on specifications later translated into the implementing acts. A practical illustration is the way public-sector and data-space catalogues in Europe commonly rely on DCAT-AP, the European application profile of the W3C DCAT vocabulary, to describe datasets consistently across portals. For health data, a specific healthcare extension was developed (HealthDataEU / HealthDCAT-AP GitLab 2025) to support catalogue requirements under EHDS (Article 77). This improves findability and comparability, but it also highlights the gap this chapter is concerned with: catalogue metadata can describe what a dataset is and where it sits, but it typically cannot carry a faithful account of how the dataset was shaped through transformations.

Within the medicines regulatory system, the Data Quality Framework for EU medicines regulation is intended to encompass primary and secondary use, as well as metadata and supporting information, e.g., master data management, underlying reference data applicable to support Committee for Medicinal Products for Human Use decision making (European Medicines Agency 2023). It generalises this logic across regulatory uses of data. It defines dimensions of data quality that include traceability, interpretability and provenance, and specifies that regulators must be able to understand the "data lifecycle", including transformations and derivations, when relying on real-world data and other complex sources for regulatory decisions. The real-world data extension to the framework reinforces that data preparation and integration steps are not neutral pre-processing but part of the evidence to be assessed.

Taken together, these instruments articulate a coherent normative picture: providers and data holders should be able to show how datasets were constructed, how potential sources of bias and error were addressed and how these choices relate to the intended context of use. From the perspective of a typical data consumer or a data engineer, however, there is a significant methodological gap. Most current systems can indicate which tables and files were used, in which environment and under which approvals, but they cannot, without substantial manual reconstruction, produce the transformation-level account that the legislation implicitly presupposes. In practice, actors respond by compiling narrative descriptions, flow diagrams and partial code excerpts that approximate the requested detail without providing a stable, computable representation of the underlying processes. The result is a latent conflict between the granularity of understanding that legal texts assume and the fragmentary nature of the artefacts that most organisations can realistically maintain under conditions of rapid iteration.

Non-European Signals and the Absence of Clear Methods

In other jurisdictions, regulatory and policy developments follow different trajectories but converge on similar expectations regarding process-level knowledge. California's Transparency in Frontier Artificial Intelligence Act (SB 53) (*SB 53*, 2025) applies to developers of "frontier models" meeting certain compute and revenue thresholds and obliges them to establish and publish a "Frontier AI framework" describing technical and organisational protocols for assessing, managing and mitigating catastrophic risks, as well as to report critical safety incidents and maintain documentation of safety measures over time. In parallel, the AI Training Data Transparency Act (AB 2013) (*AB 2013*, 2024) requires certain generative AI developers to document the provenance of training data and to disclose categories of sources used, thereby acknowledging that credible risk assessment depends on understanding how training corpora are assembled. Emerging state-level AI acts in other parts of the United States, such as the Colorado AI Act, focus on impact assessments, risk management programmes and transparency around high-risk uses, which again presuppose some structured account of data handling and model behaviour over time.

In the Gulf region, the UAE Health Data Law (Federal Law No. 2 of 2019) regulates the use of information and communication technology in healthcare and establishes a strong localisation and centralisation regime. Health data related to services provided in the UAE must, with limited exceptions, be stored, processed and generated within the state, enabling health authorities to collect, analyse and maintain health information at national level (UAE Federal Law No. 2 of 2019). The law introduces familiar data protection principles such as purpose limitation, accuracy and security and anticipates secondary uses of centrally held data for public health and planning. What it does not provide, however, is a technical vocabulary for describing how data are transformed as they move from clinical systems into national repositories and onward into analytical datasets. The emphasis lies on where data are held and under whose authority, not on how their content is reshaped.

Beyond these concrete statutes, a broader layer of soft law and model instruments is emerging. Initiatives such as the Model Law on Health Data Governance under the Transform Health coalition (*Health Data Governance—Model Law on Health Data Governance* n.d.) and regional frameworks like the African Union Data Policy Framework call for robust governance of health data, emphasising transparency, accountability and rights-based principles in data use. Academic analyses of data protection and AI governance in regions such as Africa and the Middle East reach similar conclusions: existing laws foreground consent, purpose limitation and security, but struggle to address questions arising from complex analytics and AI systems without clearer concepts for data lifecycle and transformation transparency. In these settings, just as in Europe and North America, the regulatory gaze has begun to move inside the black box of data processing, while the means of making that interior visible remain underspecified.

Structural Implication: An Implicit Demand for Process-Level Provenance

Across these different instruments, the common pattern is not a harmonised legal vocabulary but a shared structural expectation. Legislators and regulators assume that organisations can give a coherent account of how data have been assembled, transformed and used throughout the lifecycle of analytical studies and AI systems. Provisions on dataset suitability, bias mitigation and risk management presuppose insight into preprocessing, cohort construction, feature engineering and monitoring. Requirements for impact assessments, transparency reports and data quality labelling assume that relevant choices can be described and, at least in principle, revisited when systems are reassessed.

At the same time, most frameworks stop short of specifying how such process-level knowledge should be represented. Primary legislation refers to data governance, documentation and logging and often gestures towards future standards or guidance, but it does not provide a stable substrate through which the internal life of data pipelines can be conveyed in a way that is both faithful to practice and usable at scale. In response, organisations tend to produce narrative reports, diagrams and partial code extracts that approximate the requested detail without forming a systematic, portable account of transformations. Compliance becomes an exercise in assembling documents rather than in exposing processes in a structured form.

This misalignment is not only impractical, but structurally flawed. The regulation has moved into the territory of processes, while most evidentiary mechanisms remain oriented towards environments and static artefacts. Under current trajectories, the cumulative effect is an implicit demand for process-level provenance: a representation that records how data are manipulated and under which conditions, at a granularity sufficient to support the kinds of questions legal and governance frameworks now pose. The term provenance may not appear in statutory texts and where it does it is often loosely defined, but the underlying necessity is clear. Without some form of transformation-oriented, process-level record, the expectations encoded in contemporary health data and AI regulation risk remaining aspirational, because neither data users nor evaluators can reliably demonstrate or examine the behaviour that these frameworks seek to govern.

Actionable Provenance as Infrastructural Response

Transformation-Level Provenance

The developments described above suggest that the missing element in current oversight arrangements is not another layer of narrative documentation, but a representational substrate that can carry process-level information in a structured form. Transformation-level provenance is one way to characterise such a substrate. It shifts attention from the dataset as a static object to the sequence of operations through which data are reshaped.

In this view, operations applied to data are treated as discrete events. Imputations of missing values, aggregations over time or across entities, joins between tables, derivations of new variables, masking or generalisation of identifiers, filters that define cohorts and enrichments from external sources are all recorded explicitly. Each event is associated with parameters that describe how it was carried out: the imputation method and its assumptions, the time windows or grouping variables used for aggregation, the join keys, the thresholds applied to identify outliers, the criteria used for inclusion and exclusion. These events are organised into a graph that mirrors the structure of pipelines and the dependencies between steps, so that the path from source records to analytical tables can be traced systematically.

At this level, an analytical dataset is not just a table with a name and a schema. It is the endpoint of a recorded process. To understand what the dataset means, one consults the graph of transformations, not only the column descriptions. This does not require that every line of code be exposed, but it does require that the logic of how values were produced is available in a form that can be inspected without reverse-engineering scripts or notebooks.

We term provenance actionable when it is generated automatically during execution, structured for machine processing, portable across systems and sufficiently abstract to express transformation logic independently of implementation details.

Relation to Existing Machine-Readable Metadata

There is a growing ecosystem of machine-readable metadata formats for datasets, designed to support discovery, interoperability and, increasingly, responsible use. These approaches typically describe the structure of a dataset, its variables, storage locations, licences, intended use and, in some cases, aspects of its collection and curation. They make datasets easier to find, easier to cite and easier to integrate into machine learning workflows. In doing so, they represent an important step away from purely narrative descriptions towards structured documentation.

The conception of provenance developed in this book and illustrated in Part II, is complementary but operates at a different level of granularity. Existing metadata formats generally treat the dataset as a point in time: they attach rich descriptions to a given version of a dataset, but they do not aim to capture, in a systematic way, the internal life of the pipelines that produced it. Where processing is described, it is often at a high level ("cleaning", "normalisation", "harmonisation") or embedded in free text. By contrast, transformation-level provenance focuses on the evolution of data through pipelines. It seeks to record not only that cleaning occurred, but which imputations, aggregations, re-codings, exclusions and linkages were applied, with which parameters and in which order.

This distinction is not a criticism of existing machine-readable metadata. Their purpose is to make datasets more usable and interoperable, not to bear the full weight of regulatory evidence. The point is rather that the expectations emerging from health data and AI regulation concern precisely those aspects of data handling that most current metadata approaches leave implicit. Requirements to demonstrate dataset suitability, bias mitigation and appropriate data governance assume knowledge of how data were transformed, not just of where they reside and how they are licensed. Meeting these expectations under conditions of scale and diversification requires a representation that goes beyond enriched catalogue entries, towards a structured account of the transformation history itself.

Provenance as Shared Infrastructure for Interpretive Trust

For transformation-level provenance to be actionable in this sense, certain properties are essential. It must be generated as part of execution rather than reconstructed after the fact, otherwise it will inherit the selectivity and inconsistency of manual documentation. It must be structured and machine-readable, so that events and their parameters can be queried, combined and analysed systematically, rather than being embedded in free text. It must be sufficiently stable to accompany datasets as they move between systems and institutions; when a curated cohort is exported from a clinical environment to a national research infrastructure or to an external analysis platform, the associated provenance graph should travel with it in a form that remains interpretable. At the same time, it must be abstract enough to be independent of specific code and platform details, capturing the logic of transformations rather than the syntactic particulars of any one implementation.

When these conditions are met, provenance ceases to be an auxiliary log and becomes part of the infrastructure of data ecosystems. It provides a shared substrate on which different actors can base their understanding of how results were produced, even when they operate under different legal regimes, technical architectures or organisational constraints. A health data access body labelling datasets for secondary use, a regulator examining evidence in a conformity assessment and a research group reusing a cohort prepared elsewhere can all, in principle, interrogate the same graph of transformations expressed in a common semantic vocabulary. Interpretive trust no longer depends primarily on informal proximity to the original development team or on the ability to reconcile extensive narrative documentation. It depends on the quality and completeness of the recorded process history. In diversified, data-intensive health systems, such provenance becomes the medium through which claims about safety, fairness and accountability can be examined in a way that is compatible with the scale and tempo of contemporary infrastructures.

In this arrangement, provenance provides the medium through which the internal life of data pipelines becomes visible in a form that others can inspect and reason about. The Medicare use case is meant to make this concrete: provenance is not only stored, it is queryable and interpretable as a transformation history. What it does not yet provide is a way to decide, systematically and at scale, whether the recorded behaviour is acceptable in light of regulatory, ethical or methodological expectations. Once transformation histories are available as structured objects rather than as implicit traces in code and documents, part of that decision-making can in principle shift from human reconstruction to structured evaluation. The question then becomes how to express relevant conditions in a form that can be applied to provenance without collapsing the distinction between building systems and governing them or how compliance logic can be formalised and applied to structured provenance records. This question is the focus of the next chapter.

References

Cole, C., Li, S., Machin, T., Chalstrey, E., Craddock, M., Hetherington, J., Madge, J., O'Reilly, M., Robinson, J., Swanepoel, N., & Sood, H. (2023). *SATRE: Standardised Architecture for Trusted Research Environments* (Report No. Version 1.0). DARE UK (Data and Analytics Research Environments UK). https://doi.org/10.5281/zenodo.10055345

European Medicines Agency. (2023). *Data Quality Framework for EU medicines regulation* (Guideline No. EMA/326985/2023). European Medicines Agency. https://www.ema.europa.eu/en/documents/regulatory-procedural-guideline/data-quality-framework-eu-medicines-regulation_en.pdf

Generative artificial intelligence: Training data transparency (Issue AB 2013). (2024). https://legiscan.com/CA/text/AB2013/id/3023192

Health Data Governance—Model Law on Health Data Governance. (n.d.). Retrieved December 29, 2025, from https://healthdatagovernance.org/model-law/

HealthDataEU / HealthDCAT-AP · GitLab. (2025, November 7). GitLab. https://code.europa.eu/healthdataeu/healthdcat-ap

Kilian, R., Jäck, L., & Ebel, D. (2025). European AI Standards – Technical Standardisation and Implementation Challenges under the EU AI Act. *European Journal of Risk Regulation, 16*(3), 1038–1062. https://doi.org/10.1017/err.2025.10032

Mitchell, M., Wu, S., Zaldivar, A., Barnes, P., Vasserman, L., Hutchinson, B., Spitzer, E., Raji, I. D., & Gebru, T. (2019). Model Cards for Model Reporting. *Proceedings of the Conference on Fairness, Accountability, and Transparency*, 220–229. https://doi.org/10.1145/3287560.3287596

Transparency in Frontier Artificial Intelligence Act: Senate Bill 53 (Issue SB 53). (2025). https://legiscan.com/CA/text/SB53/id/3270002

Wilkinson, M. D., Dumontier, M., Aalbersberg, Ij. J., Appleton, G., Axton, M., Baak, A., Blomberg, N., Boiten, J.-W., da Silva Santos, L. B., Bourne, P. E., Bouwman, J., Brookes, A. J., Clark, T., Crosas, M., Dillo, I., Dumon, O., Edmunds, S., Evelo, C. T., Finkers, R., … Mons, B. (2016). The FAIR Guiding Principles for scientific data management and stewardship. *Scientific Data, 3*(1), 160018. https://doi.org/10.1038/sdata.2016.18

Chapter 13
From Provenance to Computable Trust

This chapter explains how transformation-level provenance can become a computable substrate for trust. Instead of reconstructing pipeline behaviour from narrative documents and scattered artefacts, organisations can evaluate recorded transformation histories using external predicates: rules expressed as queries over provenance. The chapter separates the pipeline paradigm, oriented toward utility and performance, from the compliance paradigm, oriented toward risk, obligations and safeguards and shows why a shared semantic layer is needed to connect them. It argues that "compliance-as-code" should be understood narrowly here as data-centric checks over recorded behaviour, not as an attempt to encode whole legal regimes. The chapter also shows why semantics and rule libraries must be governed as first-class objects, otherwise the burden spiral simply reappears at a higher layer. The result is a shift from episodic review toward more continuous, computable assurance, while keeping human judgement central.

After completing this chapter, readers should be able to:

- State the preconditions for computable trust from provenance: coverage and granularity, runtime capture and shared semantic typing of transformations
- Explain the architecture: pipeline paradigm vs compliance paradigm, the role of a shared semantic layer and external predicates over provenance
- Anticipate second-order risks: governance of ontologies and rule sets, update cycles, versioning and how to avoid rule proliferation recreating the burden spiral

M. Bouzinier et al., *Research Data that Can Be Trusted*,
SpringerBriefs in Computer Science, https://doi.org/10.1007/978-3-032-21032-6_13

Preconditions: From Recorded History to Computable Substrate

Provenance as More than "Better Logging"

The preceding chapter argued that the bottleneck in contemporary oversight is not the absence of information about data processes but the form in which this information is represented. Transformation-level, actionable provenance was introduced as a way of recording what is done to data in terms that expose operations, parameters and dependencies, rather than only files, tables and environments. In this view an analytical dataset is not a static object but the endpoint of a recorded process, and interpretive trust rests on the ability to interrogate that process. This already goes beyond conventional logging and lineage: it does not simply show that a pipeline ran in a particular environment under a given approval, but describes in a structured way which imputations, aggregations, exclusions, encodings and linkages shaped the content of the data. It is oriented to the questions raised by interpretive trust, not only to operational accountability.

In practice, many pipelines already contain compliance-relevant considerations, although in a form that remains opaque to those who were not involved in their development. De-identification routines, masking of identifiers, suppression of small cells, avoidance of specific joins or linkages and informal rules about which sources may be combined are routinely embedded in code and team conventions. The problem is not that the pipeline world is indifferent to regulatory and ethical constraints. It is that these constraints are entangled with implementation details, scattered across scripts and notebooks and rarely surfaced as explicit, portable objects. When evaluators seek to understand whether obligations on privacy, bias mitigation or dataset suitability have been met, they face layers of code whose implicit logic cannot be reconstructed reliably within the available time and expertise.

In this setting, the role of actionable provenance is not to replace human judgement but to rebalance where that judgement is applied. Instead of expending effort on reconstructing processes from heterogeneous artefacts, reviewers can rely on a representation that makes the internal life of pipelines visible in a stable form (PROV-DM: The PROV Data Model, 2013). The remaining question, which motivates this chapter, is how such recorded histories can be turned into evidence that can be assessed systematically and at scale.

Technical and Institutional Prerequisites

For provenance to serve as a substrate for computable trust, certain technical and institutional preconditions must be acknowledged. First, provenance capture must achieve sufficient coverage and granularity to support meaningful checks. Not every intermediate variable and configuration parameter needs to be recorded, but the events that materially affect interpretive trust—imputation of missing values, handling of rare categories, cohort restrictions, censoring, masking and enrichment with external sources—must be represented as first-class elements with identifiable parameters. Without this level of detail, many of the questions that regulation and governance now pose cannot be answered in a determinate way.

Second, these events must be annotated in a semantic vocabulary that is shared within and, eventually, across institutions. Operations such as statistical imputation, structural transformation, masking of identifiers or enrichment from external registries occur in many pipelines, but without a common categorisation evaluators cannot formulate predicates that generalise beyond individual implementations. If one team records a step as outlier handling and another as data cleaning, while a third does not distinguish it at all, rules over provenance cannot reliably detect whether particular safeguards were applied. A minimal, stable set of transformation types and attributes therefore becomes part of the infrastructure for interpretive trust (Chhetri et al. 2025).

Third, provenance capture must be integrated into execution rather than reconstructed retrospectively. When records are assembled after the fact from logs, code comments and team memory, they inherit the selectivity and inconsistency of manual documentation. Important details are omitted, intermediate states are simplified and synchrony with deployed versions is easily lost. Embedding provenance emission into runtime ensures that the recorded history corresponds to what actually happened, not to what actors recall or consider salient at the time of reporting.

These preconditions are not cost-free. Capturing fine-grained provenance might introduce overhead in execution and storage, and retrofitting existing pipelines may require substantial engineering work. At the same time, expressing transformations in a descriptive, compilable form can reduce interpretive burden and open space for consistent optimisation: provenance is generated as a by-product of declaring transformations, and the same representation can be used to standardise, test and tune execution. Agreeing on semantic categories for transformations is itself a governance task, involving data engineers, statisticians, domain experts and compliance officers. Institutions vary in their incentives and capacities to invest in such infrastructure. It is therefore important to be explicit that the move towards actionable provenance and computable trust will be incremental. Early deployments are likely to focus on priority pipelines and on a limited set of transformation types that are most relevant for risk and regulatory scrutiny. Provenance coverage and semantic maturity can then grow over time, and with them the scope of questions that can be addressed through computation rather than manual reconstruction.

Why Preconditions Are Worth Pursuing

The justification for investing in these preconditions is that the demand for provenance already exists, even when it is not named as such. Regulatory instruments in health and AI increasingly require that organisations be able to describe the lifecycle of data, explain how training, validation and test datasets were assembled, document preprocessing and curation choices and demonstrate that biases and errors have been addressed in ways appropriate to the intended use. Data quality frameworks in medicines regulation and health data governance link fitness-for-purpose to traceability of transformations and documentation of derivations. Quality management in clinical data warehouses relies on understanding how extraction, transformation and loading processes propagate or correct data issues across tables and flows. Scientific debates about reproducibility and bias in AI repeatedly return to the difficulty of understanding how datasets were prepared and which assumptions were embedded in data preparation code (Leipzig et al. 2021). In all these settings, provenance is implicitly required; it is simply provided in forms—narrative descriptions coupled to opaque code—that cannot support interpretive trust at scale.

Capturing transformation-level provenance in a structured way therefore serves multiple purposes at once. It underpins reproducibility by allowing others to re-run or re-implement workflows with a clear understanding of how data were transformed. It supports internal quality management by making error patterns and their causes traceable across pipelines. It provides a more coherent evidentiary basis for regulatory submissions than ad hoc dossiers assembled from heterogeneous artefacts. It offers a foundation on which questions about privacy, bias and representativeness can be posed in a systematic way. The effort required to emit and semantically organise provenance is thus not an additional burden layered on top of existing obligations, but a way of consolidating the representational work already demanded across scientific, operational and regulatory contexts.

Once provenance exists as a computable object, at least for critical parts of the data landscape, the central bottleneck shifts. The problem is no longer that actors do not know what happened to the data, but that they lack a structured means of deciding whether what happened is acceptable in the light of evolving obligations and safeguards. The remainder of this chapter addresses that problem by examining how external rules can be expressed and applied over provenance in a way that supports interpretive trust without recreating the burden spiral at a new layer.

Two Paradigms that Must Meet: Data Pipelines and Compliance

The Pipeline Paradigm

Data preparation pipelines are built to produce datasets that answer domain questions, under technical and organisational constraints. Their orientation is primarily towards utility and performance: extracting variables from heterogeneous sources, joining tables across systems, constructing features, training and comparing models and iterating until error metrics, stability indicators or business objectives are met.

Data engineers, statisticians, machine learning specialists and domain experts decide how to encode diagnoses, how to aggregate events over time, how to handle missingness or how to stratify cohorts, balancing model performance, interpretability for clinicians or researchers, computational cost and delivery timelines. Within this frame, a pipeline is a sequence of operations that connects raw inputs to usable outputs as efficiently and robustly as possible.

Compliance considerations are not absent from this world, but they typically appear as implicit norms rather than explicit objects. Teams may know that certain identifiers must be masked before export, that specific joins should be avoided because they increase re-identification risk, that date of birth should be generalised to year or age band or that some sources are considered out of scope for a given application. These constraints are encoded in code patterns, naming conventions and informal checklists and are transmitted through team memory and local practice rather than through a structured representation. As data engineers and analysts change roles, as pipelines evolve or are reused for new studies, this tacit mindset is fragile: it can be applied inconsistently, forgotten or overridden without leaving a trace that is visible to those outside the immediate development context.

Descriptive workflow approaches and domain-specific languages mitigate part of this opacity by lifting some aspects of pipeline logic above raw code. Instead of a collection of scripts and notebooks, they express transformations as declarative steps, emphasising the "what" over the "how". Joins, aggregations, imputations and filters are described as operators with parameters, and dependencies between steps are made explicit in the workflow definition. This already creates a metalanguage on the pipeline side: a vocabulary in which operations that matter for analytical validity can be named and related without committing to a specific implementation. Yet even where such languages are used, the link between these operations and compliance-relevant concepts remains largely implicit. The semantics of masking, enrichment or cohort restriction may be evident to the team that designs the workflow, but they are not systematically aligned with the needs of those who must assess whether legal and ethical obligations have been met.

The Compliance and Governance Paradigm

The compliance and governance paradigm arises from a different set of concerns and a different constellation of actors. Compliance officers, policy specialists within organisations, members of ethics committees, auditors, reviewers in notified bodies and staff in regulatory authorities all work with frameworks whose primary orientation is towards risk and harm avoidance, fairness, legal and ethical obligations and the maintenance of trust in institutions. Their task is to articulate what must be prevented, what must be demonstrated and which safeguards must be in place when systems handle sensitive data or influence important decisions. In this world, categories such as high-risk AI systems, vulnerable populations, sensitive attributes, proportionality and necessity structure how data processing is judged. Thresholds, prohibitions and required safeguards are defined: maximum tolerable error rates in particular settings, limits on the use of certain data types, mandatory documentation of validation and monitoring, obligations to detect and mitigate bias, constraints on secondary uses and reuse. Justifications play a central role. Actors are expected to explain why a given dataset is suitable for its intended purpose, why certain transformations are appropriate, why residual risks are acceptable and how they are controlled over time.

These compliance artefacts are predominantly textual and institutional. They include legal acts, regulatory guidelines, professional standards, internal policies, codes of conduct and ethics board opinions. Templates for impact assessments, risk registers, data management plans, data quality frameworks and audit reports translate these norms into structured but still narrative forms. They ask for descriptions of data sources, purposes, categories of data subjects, processing operations, safeguards, residual risks and mitigation measures. Increasingly, they also request accounts of training, validation and test data, preprocessing steps, feature construction, monitoring regimes and update procedures. All these instruments presuppose insight into the processes that shape data and model behaviour, yet they are written for human interpretation and rely on manual translation into practice by the various experts involved.

This reliance has practical consequences. When organisations respond to these requirements, they assemble documentation that mirrors the structure of the templates and legal texts rather than the structure of their pipelines. They describe sources and purposes, outline high-level processing steps and summarise validation results, but they rarely express, in a stable and machine-readable form, how specific transformations relate to specific obligations. The connection between a prohibition on using a particular attribute as a predictor and the code that implements feature engineering remains mediated by human judgement and local understanding, whether on the side of internal compliance teams or external auditors. As long as this is the case, compliance logic cannot be applied directly to recorded behaviour; it must be interpreted and manually mapped onto the artefacts that pipelines produce.

Semantic Alignment as a Shared Middle Layer

Both worlds ultimately refer to the same underlying processes. When a data engineer talks about imputing missing values in a variable, collapsing categories in a diagnosis code or enriching a dataset with external registry information, and when a regulator, auditor or ethics committee member asks whether missingness was handled appropriately, whether rare conditions were excluded in a way that introduces bias or whether external data sources were authorised and suitable, they are pointing to the same operations. The divergence lies in the vocabularies used and in the forms in which these operations are represented. If provenance is to serve as a substrate for computable trust, a shared semantic layer is needed in which these processes can be named and related in a way that both worlds can understand.

This layer consists of types of transformations and their attributes, expressed in a controlled yet extensible vocabulary. Categories such as statistical imputation, suppression and masking of identifiers, cohort restriction, enrichment with external data, derivation of composite indicators, application of particular algorithms or models and monitoring of drift become explicit objects. Each recorded event in a provenance graph is not only an execution of an operator in a given workflow language but also an instance of one or more of these semantic categories, with parameters that matter for governance: imputation method and rate, masking strategy, inclusion and exclusion criteria, source and version of external data, algorithm identifier and its approval status, trigger and outcome of monitoring procedures.

The crucial requirement is that pipeline metalanguages and compliance metalanguages both point to this shared layer. On the pipeline side, workflow descriptions and DSL operators must be mapped to transformation categories in a way that is stable enough for internal validation teams, external auditors and regulators to rely on. On the governance side, rules-as-code and other structured representations of obligations must express their conditions in terms of the same categories and attributes. Only then can automated evaluation of provenance become meaningful. Without such alignment, predicates would either be too vague to be operationalised or too tightly bound to particular implementations to be reusable. Establishing and maintaining this semantic middle layer is therefore not a marginal technical detail but a central element in making the interaction between pipeline work and compliance work computable.

External Predicates over Provenance: Compliance-as-Code in a Narrow Sense

What It Means to Run Rules over Provenance

Once transformation-level provenance is available as a structured graph, it becomes possible to ask determinate questions about recorded behaviour without re-entering the pipeline code (O'Sullivan et al. 2025). Predicates over provenance can be understood as machine-readable statements that query this graph and return well-defined answers: a Boolean value, a count, a range of values or a set of identified events (*Philosophy| Open Policy Agent*, n.d.). They are formulated in terms of the semantic categories and attributes introduced in the previous section, not in terms of the internal syntax of any particular workflow language. We further explore this approach in Appendix B discussing a DSL example for policy makers and governance experts.

Typical questions illustrate the scope. One class concerns the extent and manner of imputation. A predicate might ask whether imputation for a given variable exceeded an agreed proportion of records in the dataset, or whether specific methods were used where they are known to be inappropriate. Another class concerns the treatment of subgroups. Predicates can be formulated to detect whether individuals in a defined subgroup, such as a particular age category or minority population, were systematically excluded by a sequence of filters, or whether their representation fell below a threshold that had been set as a safeguard against unrecognised bias.

Further predicates address the handling of sensitive attributes. They can be used to verify that a given attribute was only used in contexts that had been explicitly authorised, or that it did not enter the feature set for a predictive model where its use would be considered discriminatory. Similar checks can be defined for data sources and algorithms. A predicate can confirm that a specified registry or external dataset was not used to construct an outcome label where this would create circularity, or that a family of algorithms designated as non-compliant for a particular application did not appear in the recorded transformations. Finally, predicates can be attached to monitoring and lifecycle management. They can verify that a retraining or monitoring pipeline was executed when a drift indicator exceeded a defined threshold, that the resulting evaluation was recorded and that an appropriate response was triggered. In each case, the predicate does not infer behaviour from documentation; it reads it from the provenance graph.

The account that follows should be read as a conceptual pattern rather than as a description of a specific implementation. Different technical stacks can realise predicates in different ways, but the underlying idea is the same: once provenance encodes what has been done to data in a structured form, part of the evidentiary work can in principle be expressed as queries over that structure.

Externality and Division of Labour

In this pattern, predicates do not prescribe how pipelines must be written. They operate on recorded behaviour after the fact, interpreting what has actually been done to the data. Their function is to evaluate whether the history captured in provenance satisfies a set of conditions derived from regulatory, ethical or methodological expectations. The design of pipelines and the design of predicates are therefore distinct activities, even if they must be coordinated. Recent research has explored the use of predicates to constrain self-modifying AI systems so that they maintain specific safety properties (Bukatin 2024), but similar predicate-based constraints could likewise be imposed on pipelines engineered by humans.

On one side, those who design and operate pipelines focus on analytical questions. They define workflows, choose algorithms, adjust parameters and manage performance, and as part of execution their systems emit provenance events annotated with the agreed semantic categories. The primary concern at this stage is that provenance be complete and accurate enough to support later evaluation, not that it anticipates every possible rule that might be applied.

On the other side, those responsible for compliance and oversight define and maintain predicates that evaluate provenance against obligations and safeguards. They identify which conditions are sufficiently clear, stable and important to warrant formalisation, and they express these conditions as queries over the provenance model. The same group interprets predicate outcomes: deciding, for example, whether a marginal breach of a threshold is acceptable in context, or whether repeated violations signal a structural problem in how pipelines are designed.

This division of labour mirrors experience in systems that already distinguish between internal analytical logic and external statements about that logic. In some clinical genomics platforms, for example, the rules that define which variants are considered relevant for a diagnostic hypothesis are separate from statements that describe properties of those rules, such as the domains of knowledge they rely on or the conditions under which they should be updated. The predicate layer over provenance generalises this pattern. The transformations that constitute a data preparation pipeline correspond to the internal logic, while predicates express statements that must hold about this logic if certain obligations are to be met. Keeping these layers separate reduces the risk that pipelines become entangled with local interpretations of regulation and allows compliance reasoning to evolve without requiring constant modification of analytical code.

Compliance-as-Code without "coding the law"

The approach described here fits within broader discussions of compliance-as-code and policy-as-code, but in a deliberately narrow sense. The aim is not to encode entire regulatory regimes in software or to replace legal judgement with automated decision-making. This aligns with the direction signalled by the OECD's call in 2020 for "rulemaking for humans and machines" (Mohun and Roberts 2020): governance that can operate at scale requires rules expressed in forms that both people and systems can interpret. Most provisions governing health data and AI systems are too open-textured, context-dependent and value-laden to be reduced to executable rules without serious distortion; the goal is therefore more modest and more specific: to formalise selected obligations and safeguards that lend themselves to precise, data-linked checks and that are already implicit in current practice.

Many of the example predicates correspond directly to expectations formulated in recent instruments. Requirements that training, validation and test data be appropriate, representative and subject to documented preprocessing and bias mitigation measures, or that real-world data used for regulatory purposes be traceable across their lifecycle, imply questions about imputation rates, exclusion patterns and enrichment steps that can be expressed over provenance. Obligations to monitor model performance and address drift imply questions about whether monitoring pipelines were executed when conditions were met and whether outcomes were acted upon. Provisions that restrict the use of particular data types or sources in certain contexts, or that require transparency about the provenance of training corpora, can be supported by predicates that verify the absence or controlled presence of specified attributes, registries or datasets in the recorded transformations.

Formulating such predicates does not exhaust the evidentiary burden associated with these frameworks, but it can address a significant part of it. Instead of requiring reviewers to infer from narrative descriptions and scattered technical artefacts whether an obligation has been met, a subset of questions can be answered by computation over provenance graphs. This does not obviate the need for human interpretation; the meaning and sufficiency of predicate outcomes remain matters for judgement. It does, however, change the structure of the volume crisis described earlier. Where provenance and a carefully governed set of predicates are available, the marginal cost of answering recurring questions about data handling becomes low, and the answers become more consistent across systems and institutions. Human attention can then be focused on aspects that resist formalisation and on cases where predicate evaluations indicate that behaviour is close to, or has crossed, agreed boundaries.

Governing Semantics and Rules: Avoiding a Second Burden Spiral

The Risk of Semantic and Rule Overload

A semantic layer for transformations and a predicate layer for compliance create new objects that themselves require governance. Deciding what counts as imputation, masking, cohort restriction or enrichment is not neutral. If every project or institution defines its own categories, the same operation will be labelled differently across systems and provenance will cease to be comparable.

Once predicates over provenance are available, rules can also proliferate. Different groups may add checks in response to internal policies, audits or specific incidents. Without coordination, rules overlap, conflict and persist after their rationale has faded.

If left unmanaged, these dynamics recreate the burden spiral at a new layer. Provenance may make transformations visible, yet evaluation becomes opaque again because semantics are local and rule sets are dense and inconsistent. External validators would have to learn each institution's ontology and rule history before they can interpret a provenance graph. Avoiding this outcome requires treating semantics and predicates as explicit governance objects (Chhetri et al. 2025).

Principles for Governing Semantics

The semantic layer should evolve under clear constraints. First, scope should be modest. A small core vocabulary of transformation types is sufficient to start: imputation of missing values, masking or generalisation of identifiers, cohort restriction, enrichment from external sources, derivation of composite indicators, application of model families and execution of monitoring or retraining procedures. Finer distinctions can be added when repeated use cases justify them.

Second, extensions should follow a change process with versioning and attention to backwards compatibility. When a new category is introduced or an existing one refined, its relation to the previous vocabulary and its impact on existing provenance and predicates should be recorded.

Third, semantics should be openly documented. Definitions of transformation types, their attributes and example mappings from common workflow languages should be available so that other tools and institutions can align or define explicit mappings. Predicates do not operate on arbitrary function names but on this deliberately defined ontology of transformation types. Only operations mapped to these types, with agreed attributes, become visible to the rule layer.

In practice, such vocabularies rarely emerge from abstract negotiation. They crystallise around working systems that already need a computable classification of evidence or transformations. Our earlier work presented at Bioinformatics Open Source Conference in 2025 (Etin et al. 2025) on structured evidence ontologies in variant interpretation shows that constrained, purpose-built vocabularies can support both machine reasoning and human review. A similar pattern can be followed here: platforms and workflow languages that emit transformation-level provenance publish a reference ontology; others adopt it, adapt it or map their local categories to it. Over time, as multiple infrastructures converge on similar patterns, these vocabularies can be taken up by communities around trusted research environments and health data spaces and, where appropriate, feed into formal standardisation. The immediate aim is not a single global standard, but a small number of widely understood baselines that make provenance interpretable across institutional boundaries.

Principles for Governing Rule Sets

The predicate layer benefits from the same discipline. Rules should be treated as a curated library, not as an unbounded list of checks. This implies clarity on stewardship (who can propose, approve and retire rules), explicit scope (which pipelines, datasets or applications a predicate applies to) and mechanisms to detect and resolve conflicts where obligations differ across domains or jurisdictions.

Predicates should also have a lifecycle. New rules can be introduced on a trial basis, observed in practice, refined and eventually deprecated when frameworks change or when they no longer add value. Maintaining a catalogue that records the rationale, scope and status of predicates keeps the rule landscape intelligible and avoids silent accumulation. Under such conditions, a limited set of well-understood, high-value predicates can reduce the interpretive burden rather than add to it.

Net Benefit: Why the Additional Structure Is Worth it

Governing semantics and rules entails real overhead. Experts must agree on categories, maintain mappings and curate rule sets. The case for this effort rests on the way provenance and predicates function as shared infrastructure. Once a core ontology and a curated rule library exist, each additional check is cheap to execute and reusable across runs, studies and submissions.

The same structures serve several purposes at once: internal quality management, scientific reproducibility, regulatory evidence and institutional governance rely on the same provenance graphs and predicates. Effort shifts from repeatedly recreating narrative descriptions of similar processes to maintaining shared representations and checks that many actors can rely on. Under regulatory and ethical expectations that already require an account of how data are transformed, this shift is not an extra burden but a way to make those expectations compatible with data-intensive infrastructures.

From Episodic Review to Continuous, Computable Assurance

Changing the Practice of Oversight

If provenance becomes a routine output of data preparation pipelines and predicates over provenance are in place, the practice of oversight can move from episodic review to continuous assurance. Today, formal interactions between operators and oversight bodies are organised around dossiers: assembled at specific points in time, tailored to particular frameworks and largely narrative in form. Much of the effort on both sides is spent reconstructing what was done to data and mapping recurring questions onto heterogeneous artefacts.

In a provenance- and predicate-based model, the primary evidentiary object is the recorded history of data transformations, expressed in a shared semantic vocabulary, together with the outcomes of agreed checks on that history. Rules can be evaluated after each execution, periodically across families of runs or when specific events occur, such as the introduction of a new data source or a model update. Evidence for compliance becomes a by-product of routine operation rather than a separate reporting exercise. Episodic reviews do not disappear, but they draw on a standing layer of computable evidence instead of starting from reconstruction each time. Oversight shifts from reading pipelines through documents to examining rule outcomes and investigating exceptions.

In this narrow, data-centric sense, part of compliance becomes automated. What is being automated is not regulatory judgement but a layer of recurring interpretive work: checking whether concrete data processes meet clearly formulated conditions that can be linked back to obligations on privacy, bias control, data quality and lifecycle governance.

The New Role of Human Judgement

Automating this layer does not diminish the role of human judgement; it repositions it. People decide which obligations and safeguards merit formalisation as predicates and which must remain in narrative, deliberative or case-based form. They interpret predicate results, distinguish between benign deviations and signals of structural problems and investigate the causes of failures where checks indicate that conditions are not met. They adapt semantics and rule sets when technical practice, legal requirements or ethical expectations change.

Many questions at the heart of trust in health data systems resist precise formalisation. Contextual fairness, the acceptability of residual risks, the distribution of benefits and burdens across populations and the broader legitimacy of particular uses of data are political and ethical matters. Computable trust does not attempt to resolve them. Its contribution is to provide a more stable evidentiary base: when disagreements arise about whether a system is acceptable, actors can refer to an inspectable account of what has been done to data, which safeguards fired or failed to fire and how these relate to explicit expectations, rather than to partial reconstructions assembled under time pressure.

Closing: A New Form of Delegated Understanding

In this part we have argued that sustaining trust in data-intensive health systems requires reconfiguring both how we record data processes and how we evaluate them. Chapters 10 and 11 showed that human-bounded trust mechanisms reach structural limits when systems generate more evidentiary material than reviewers can absorb and when oversight operates at a distance from the pipelines it must judge. Adding further documentation and guidance under these conditions produces the burden spiral rather than deeper understanding.

Chapter 12 reframed this as a problem of representation and introduced transformation-level provenance as the missing substrate: a way of recording what is done to data, oriented to interpretive trust and compatible with scale. This chapter added the evaluative mechanism: external predicates over that provenance, expressed in a shared semantic layer and governed as curated rule sets, together with principles for managing their evolution so that they do not recreate overload. In this configuration, compliance-as-code acquires a specific, limited meaning. It is not an attempt to encode whole regulatory regimes, but a way to express selected, data-linked obligations as computable conditions on recorded transformations.

This raises questions that we can only frame, not fully answer. How far can formalisation of this kind go before it distorts the underlying norms it is meant to support. Which institutions should act as stewards of shared semantics and rule libraries, and how can their authority be made accountable. How will differences between regulatory regimes and local practices be reflected in predicates without fragmenting the common substrate needed for cross-border research and regulation. And how will power asymmetries between large actors, who can shape de facto standards and smaller institutions, who must adopt them, be managed.

What can be stated with some confidence is that trust in data-intensive health systems will increasingly depend on how well we can represent data processes and subject those representations to structured, computable checks, without losing sight of the political and ethical questions they cannot decide. Provenance and compliance-as-code, in the restricted sense developed here, offer a new way of delegating understanding: from individuals to representations and from representations to governed rule sets. This form of delegated understanding is more compatible with the scale, speed and diversity of contemporary infrastructures than purely narrative mechanisms, but it depends on sustained investment in shared semantics and disciplined rule governance.

Parts I and II of this book address the technical realisation of this architecture: the design of dataflow operators and domain-specific languages that emit transformation-level provenance, and their implementation in concrete platforms and pipelines. Part IV provides a classification of data transformations that can serve as a starting point for the shared semantic layer discussed in this chapter. Together, these parts show that the conceptual requirements outlined here are not merely aspirational but can be approximated in working systems, with the compromises and limitations that practical deployment entails.

References

Bukatin, M. (2024). *Pondering Invariant Properties of Self-Modifying Systems*. https://doi.org/10.13140/RG.2.2.19271.15523

Chhetri, T. R., Halchenko, Y. O., Jarecka, D., Trivedi, P., Ghosh, S. S., Ray, P., & Ng, L. (2025). Bridging the Scientific Knowledge Gap and Reproducibility: A Survey of Provenance, Assertion and Evidence Ontologies. *Companion Proceedings of the ACM on Web Conference 2025*, 924–928. https://doi.org/10.1145/3701716.3715483

Etin, D., Bouzinier, M., Trifonov, S., Lvova, E., Shavtvalishvili, G., & Chmuack, M. (2025). Formal validation of variant classification rules using domain-specific language and meta-predicates. *F1000Research, 14*. https://doi.org/10.7490/f1000research.1120271.1

Leipzig, J., Nüst, D., Hoyt, C. T., Ram, K., & Greenberg, J. (2021). The role of metadata in reproducible computational research. *Patterns, 2*(9). https://doi.org/10.1016/j.patter.2021.100322

Mohun, J., & Roberts, A. (2020). *Cracking the Code: Rulemaking for Humans and Machines* (OECD Working Papers on Public Governance No. 42). Organisation for Economic Co-operation and Development (OECD). https://doi.org/10.1787/3afe6ba5-en

O'Sullivan, K., Markovic, M., Dymiter, J., Scheliga, B., Odo, C., & Wilde, K. (2025). Semi-automated data provenance tracking for transparent data production and linkage to enhance auditing and quality assurance in Trusted Research Environments. *International Journal of Population Data Science, 10*(2). https://doi.org/10.23889/ijpds.v10i2.2464

Philosophy | Open Policy Agent. (n.d.). Retrieved December 29, 2025, from https://openpolicyagent.org/docs/philosophy

PROV-DM: The PROV Data Model (W3C Recommendation No. PROV-DM). (2013). World Wide Web Consortium (W3C). https://www.w3.org/TR/prov-dm/

Part IV
Classification of Data Transformations

Chapter 14
A Taxonomy of Data Transformations

This chapter revisits and substantially extends the brief taxonomy of data transformations introduced in Chap. 5. Whereas Chap. 5 focused on giving readers enough intuition to follow the platform design, here we aim at a more complete and formal classification for readers who will design or implement provenance-aware data-modelling DSLs.

After completing this chapter, readers should be able to:

- Distinguish between isomorphic and non-isomorphic single-value transformations and explain how reversibility (or its absence) affects data provenance and reproducibility.
- Describe normalization and rollups, identify when each is appropriate and assess the trade-offs between canonical representation and information loss.
- Explain union transformations and datatype casting and apply them to harmonize heterogeneous datasets (e.g., multi-year or multi-source tables with differing schemas).
- Characterize approximation operators used to infer or impute missing or ambiguous values and reason about their impact on bias, uncertainty and auditability.
- Differentiate simple aggregations from custom aggregations, including the role of disambiguation rules when a single "canonical" value must be chosen from conflicting inputs.
- Describe and use operators for flattening and unnesting arrays, collapsing multiple columns into arrays and transposing columns into rows and understand how they reshape schemas.
- Analyze how each class of transformation (normalization, rollups, aggregations, approximations, unions, reshaping) influences the construction of column- and cell-level lineage.
- Apply this taxonomy of transformations when designing or extending a data-modelling DSL, selecting appropriate operator primitives and metadata needed for fine-grained provenance.

M. Bouzinier et al., *Research Data that Can Be Trusted*,
SpringerBriefs in Computer Science, https://doi.org/10.1007/978-3-032-21032-6_14

Table 14.1 Isomorphic transformation

Input dataset(s)	Input value	Output	Processing method	Reversible?
Single dataset	Single value	Single value	Arbitrary function or expression written in a procedural language, or as a valid SQL expression	Yes

Isomorphic Transformations

Isomorphic transformations are the simplest form of data transformations, where each value is converted into another in a reversible manner. This means there exists a reverse transformation that can precisely reconstruct the original value from the transformed one.

Examples:

- **State Codes Conversion**: Transforming state abbreviations (e.g., CA for California) into Federal Information Processing Standards (FIPS) codes or Social Security Administration (SSA) codes.
- **Date Format Conversion**: Converting dates from the SAS software format to the International Organization for Standardization (ISO) 8601 date format (*ISO - ISO 8601—Date and Time Format* 2017).

Transformation Characteristics (Table 14.1):

Non-isomorphic Single Value Transformations

Non-isomorphic single value transformations are used when a simplified or altered representation of the original data are sufficient for downstream analysis, despite some inherent loss of detail. These transformations are prevalent in fields that require data compression, privacy-preserving mechanisms and efficient data querying.

Examples:

- **String Truncation**: Often used to fit data into fixed-width fields or simplify data storage.
- **Hashing** (e.g., MD5): Common in creating unique, irreversible identifiers for sensitive data to protect privacy.
- **Text Summarization**: Helps in reducing detailed text information into concise summaries for quick understanding or processing.

There are several important subcases of non-isomorphic single value transformations that deserve to be considered separate type of transformations:

- Normalization
- Rollups

Table 14.2 Non-isomorphic transformation

Input dataset(s)	Input value	Output	Processing method	Reversible?
Single dataset	Single value	Single value	Arbitrary function or expression written in a procedural language, or as a valid SQL expression	No, involves loss of information

Transformation Characteristics (Table 14.2):

Normalization

Normalization is a reduction of a value to a commonly perceived canonical form. Normalization aids in creating a standard baseline for data, facilitating comparison and analysis by ensuring uniformity across datasets. It often reduces variability that can obscure true patterns in data, thus enhancing the reliability of analytical insights.

While we do not sacrifice any substantial or relevant information doing normalization, technically we incur an information loss. When we know only normalized form we have no way of knowing what was the exact original value.

Examples:

- **Transforming All Letters to Lowercase**: Common in text processing to ensure consistent search and comparison operations.
- **Genetic Variant Representation Normalization**: Mapping locally defined variant descriptions into a canonical, machine-readable form (e.g. GA4GH VRS objects), including consistent coordinate systems and left-/right-trimming rules, so that biologically equivalent variants receive the same representation and identifiers across laboratories, EHRs, research systems and knowledge bases.
- **Temperature Conversion**: Used in scientific data integration to ensure compatibility and precision in multi-source data analysis. Sometimes original temperature values can be in different units, like centigrades, degrees Fahrenheit. A common practice would be to convert all to Kelvins.
- **Normalization of date and time** to ISO form (see Isomorphic Transformations).

Rollups

Rollups are a form of data transformation that summarize or aggregate detailed data into broader categories or higher levels of abstraction reducing data granularity. They typically utilize a many-to-one mapping function, transforming input data from a single dataset. Mathematically, rollups can often be viewed as a projection from a high-dimensional space to a low-dimensional space, a form of dimensionality

Table 14.3 Rollups

Input dataset(s)	Input value	Output	Processing method	Reversible?
Single dataset	Single value	Single value	Mapping many-to-one function	No (loss of information)

reduction. By providing a concise representation of complex data, rollups facilitate easier data exploration and enhance the clarity of visualizations. They also improve the efficiency of training classification models by minimizing data clutter.

Key Examples of Rollups:

- **Extracting Temporal Components**: Simplifying a timestamp to just a date or extracting the year from a complete date-time stamp.
- **Geographic Aggregation**: Mapping specific county FIPS codes to larger geographical regions like states.
- **Medical Terminology Mapping**: Mapping specific International Classification of Diseases (ICD) codes to broader Charlson Comorbidity Index (CCI) conditions (Glasheen et al. 2019), or mapping of a SNOMED CT (*SNOMED CT United States Edition* n.d.) term to a broader term, e.g., *Peripheral arterial occlusive disease* (399957001) to *Disorder by body site* (123946008)
- **Semantic Generalization**: Mapping of a semantic type to a more general semantic type, e.g., *Antibiotic* to a *Chemical Viewed Functionally.*

Rollups serve as powerful tools for reducing data complexity while preserving essential information for analysis, however they result in a loss of some detailed information, which is a trade-off for achieving a streamlined and manageable data form.

Transformation Characteristics (Table 14.3):

Union Transformations

Union transformations are employed when combining data from multiple datasets into a unified dataset. This process is particularly necessary when consolidating data spanning multiple years into a single dataset. Union transformations should effectively handle situations where the same fields (e.g., columns) have different names or data types across various datasets. For instance, an integer field might be represented as a string in certain years, and dates could be expressed in various formats. To address these challenges and create a cohesive dataset, the data manipulation Domain-Specific Language (DSL) must provide mechanisms to:

- **Define Input Dataset Patterns**: Specify patterns to identify which datasets to include or exclude in the union process.

Table 14.4 Union transformation

Input dataset(s)	Input value	Output	Processing method	Reversible?
Multiple datasets	Single value	Single value	Field alignment, type casting and copying	Yes

- **Align Source Property Names**: Establish a pattern or list that maps output property in the combined dataset to its corresponding names across the source datasets.
- **Standardize Datatypes**: Apply rules to convert or cast properties of varying data types to a consistent datatype in the unified dataset.

Example: Combining Medicare Enrollment Records Across Multiple Years.

- Datasource Pattern:
  - Include: "mbsf_ab*"
  - Exclude: "mbsf_abcd_2021"
- Source Property List:
  - Align fields such as [dob, bene_dob, bene_birth_dt] to a unified property like "date_of_birth."
- Type Conversion Rules:
  - String to Date: parse_date({column_name})
  - Numeric to Date: to_date(to_char({column_name}, '00000000'), 'YYYYMMDD')

Transformation Characteristics (Table 14.4):

Approximations

Approximation techniques are primarily used to address problems related to missing or incomplete data. These methods help estimate the most likely values for missing data points, enabling data analysis despite data gaps.

Example:

One common use case is inferring a county FIPS code from a ZIP code or ZCTA code. While most ZIP codes fall entirely within a single county, there are exceptions. In the cases reviewed, approximately 90% of a ZIP code area typically resides within one county. Thus, using approximation techniques, it is possible to infer the county code with relatively high accuracy, though some estimations may prove incorrect due to the inherent limitations of the data.

Approximation involves the application of arbitrary functions to estimate missing values, which may not be reversible due to potential information loss in the process.

Table 14.5 Approximation

Input dataset(s)	Input value	Output	Processing method	Reversible?
Single dataset	Single value	Single or multiple value(s)	Arbitrary function	No (possible loss of information)

Table 14.6 Simple aggregation

Input dataset(s)	Input value	Output	Processing method	Reversible?
Single dataset	Multiple values	Single value	Built-in aggregation function	No

Transformation Characteristics (Table 14.5):

Simple Aggregations

Simple aggregations represent the most basic form of multi-value transformation, where multiple input values are condensed into a single output value. Generic SQL provides a variety of aggregation functions, with specific DBMSs extending these options through additional proprietary aggregations. Moreover, third-party contributions have expanded the range of available aggregations. In practice, we frequently utilize functions such as MIN, MAX, COUNT, string aggregation (creating a comma-separated list of values) and ARRAY aggregation. For string and array aggregations, DISTINCT values are often important.

Certain extensions to standard SQL aggregation are necessary within the data transformation DSL (Domain-Specific Language). For instance, COUNT(DISTINCT) may need to ignore NULL values. While this requirement is not easily captured by standard SQL, it must be expressible within the DSL.

Aggregations are inherently non-reversible, as they summarize multiple data points into a singular value, resulting in the loss of individual data details. Simple aggregations form the foundational building block for more advanced data transformation techniques, including custom aggregations and the application of disambiguation rules, which will be discussed in subsequent sections.

Transformation Characteristics (Table 14.6):

Aggregations: Disambiguation Rules

Aggregations often require disambiguation rules, particularly when the expected output is a single value but the aggregation results in a set of multiple, potentially conflicting values. Such scenarios necessitate specific disambiguation rules, which should be expressible within the data transformation DSL.

Example:

For each Medicare beneficiary, for certain data points like date of birth (DOB), sex, race, ethnicity and date of death (DOD) we expect a single value per field. However, discrepancies often arise in enrollment records, necessitating a strategy for handling such ambiguities. When it happens, the rule raises the ambiguity flag that can be recorded along with the data. Here are some disambiguation rules for managing these variances:

- **DOB**: Select the earliest DOB from the enrollment records for the primary value. Additionally, track the latest DOB as a secondary value in a separate column, setting it to NULL when DOB is unambiguous.

  From the data analyzed between 1999 and 2018, approximately 0.27% of beneficiaries exhibited ambiguous DOBs. Typically, excluding these beneficiaries from datasets is advisable unless necessary to include them—where recording the latest DOB aids in age verification.

  Most discrepancies arise from minor errors (e.g., within 10 days) or errors in the month or year, likely due to paperwork mistakes. Mismatches not aligning with these patterns may indicate the mixing of records from distinct beneficiaries.
- **DOD**: The rule is similar to DOB disambiguation but excludes NULLs from aggregations, as DOD is naturally NULL for records dated prior to a beneficiary's death. The actual rule is: select the latest recorded DOD and document the earliest DOD separately.
- **Race, ethnicity and sex**: use string aggregation for distinct values. However, adoption of more refined rules may be necessary based on user feedback. For instance, if a value is consistent across all but one enrollment year, it might be practical to default to the prevailing value, treating anomalies as artefacts. DSL should allow for such configurations, including setting thresholds on allowable record variances.

Custom Aggregations

Aggregation is generally defined as a function applied to a set of elements, summarizing them into a singular value or representation. Simple built-in aggregations, such as 'COUNT', 'SUM', 'MINIMUM', 'MAXIMUM' and 'MEAN' values, illustrate the basic possibilities. However, more complex aggregations, such as weighted or spatial aggregations, can also be employed to address specific analytical needs. In some cases, even more sophisticated algorithms are required to capture the nuances of the data. Custom aggregation is a user-defined function that maps a set of elements to a summary result.

The capacity to define user-specific aggregation functions is a significant asset in data science. This flexibility allows analysts to tailor aggregations to the unique characteristics of their datasets and analytic goals. Many database management systems (DBMS) support user-defined aggregations through plugins or custom functions.

Table 14.7 Custom aggregation

Input dataset(s)	Input value	Output	Processing method	Reversible?
Single dataset	Multiple values	Single value	User provided aggregation function	No

Ideally, a Domain-Specific Language (DSL) for data manipulation should also facilitate the definition of custom aggregations, thereby expanding analytical capabilities and precision.

Although custom aggregations are non-reversible due to their summarizing nature, they provide analysts with tools to manipulate and interpret complex datasets beyond the scope of standard aggregation functions.

Example: One example of a custom aggregation is the HyperLogLog algorithm (Heule et al. 2013) for cardinality estimation, also known as approximate `COUNT DISTINCT`. Implementations of this algorithm are available for major DBMSs and can significantly improve performance when estimating the number of distinct elements in large datasets.

Transformation Characteristics (Table 14.7):

Flattening and Unnesting of Arrays

Flattening arrays is a distinct type of aggregation. Unlike the majority of aggregations, it is reversible. The key distinction is that the resulting value is a collection (array) containing all individual elements, enabling a reverse transformation. In many DBMSs, flattening is performed using the ARRAY_AGG aggregation function.

Unnesting arrays reverses the flattening process. It maps a single record (row) with an array value in one field (column) to multiple rows, each containing a single element of the array in the corresponding column.

These transformations are well-supported by SQL, thus they do not require specialized functionality within a Domain-Specific Language (DSL).

Transformation Characteristics (Table 14.8):

Table 14.8 Arrayflattening

Transformation	Input dataset	Input value	Output	Processing method	Reversible?
Flattening	Single dataset	Multiple values	Single value	Built-in aggregation function	Yes
Unnesting	Single dataset	Single value	Multiple values	Unnest function	Yes

Collapsing Multiple Columns

Data are often uniformly distributed across several columns, complicating querying as it requires repeated conditions across each column. In some cases, it's beneficial to collapse multiple columns into an array, while in others, transposing columns into rows is more appropriate.

Examples:

- **Collapsing into Arrays**: for data like diagnosis codes in Medicare and Medicaid admissions, columns (e.g., icd_code1, icd_code2, ..., up to icd_codeN) can vary yearly, sometimes totaling up to 25. Here, the most efficient approach is collapsing all diagnosis columns into a single column of type *array*.
- **Transposing to Rows**: monthly eligibility data presents a different scenario. The Master Beneficiary Summary File (MBSF) for 2018, for instance, includes numerous parameters with data across 12 months, leading to over 500 columns. In this case, transposing these columns into rows, creating a record for each month, is advantageous.

Collapsing Multiple Columns into Arrays

This operation is straightforward yet may require boilerplate code. To simplify and streamline the process, the DSL should support wildcards or regular expressions for column names. It is often useful to combine collapsing with isomorphic transformations. For instance, when collapsing diagnoses into an array, maintain the primary diagnosis in a separate column while storing both primary and additional diagnoses within an array type column. This transformation should be clearly expressible in the data manipulation DSL.

Transformation Characteristics (Table 14.9):

Table 14.9 Collapsing columns into arrays

Input dataset(s)	Input value	Output	Processing method	Reversible?
Single dataset	Multiple values (horizontal)	Single value (array)	Combine into an array	Yes

Table 14.10 Transposing

Input dataset(s)	Input value	Output	Processing method	Reversible?
Single dataset	Multiple values (horizontal)	Multiple values (vertical)	Combine into an array and unnest	Yes

Transposing Columns to Rows

For transposing columns, the technical process involves combining columns into arrays followed by unnesting these arrays into rows. A properly designed DSL should allow a clear definition of this operation including wildcard support for column names.

Transformation Characteristics (Table 14.10):

References

Glasheen, W. P., Cordier, T., Gumpina, R., Haugh, G., Davis, J., & Renda, A. (2019). Charlson Comorbidity Index: ICD-9 Update and ICD-10 Translation. *American Health & Drug Benefits*, *12*(4), 188–197.

Heule, S., Nunkesser, M., & Hall, A. (2013). HyperLogLog in practice: Algorithmic engineering of a state of the art cardinality estimation algorithm. *Proceedings of the 16th International Conference on Extending Database Technology*, 683–692. https://doi.org/10.1145/2452376.2452456.

ISO - ISO 8601—Date and time format. (2017, February 21). ISO. https://www.iso.org/iso-8601-date-and-time-format.html

SNOMED CT United States Edition. (n.d.). [Product, Program, and Project Descriptions]. U.S. National Library of Medicine. Retrieved October 12, 2024, from https://www.nlm.nih.gov/healthit/snomedct/us_edition.html

Conclusion

Human-bounded oversight of data-intensive health systems has reached its structural limits. The mechanisms that societies developed to sustain trust in complex technical processes, documentation written for human interpretation and review conducted within the cognitive and organisational capacities of institutions, cannot absorb the volume and granularity of evidence that modern data pipelines produce. This is not a future risk but a present condition. Regulatory expectations and data preparation complexity are spiralling together: each expansion of governance scope generates more documentation demands, while each increase in pipeline sophistication produces artefacts that resist human interpretation. We described this dynamic as a volume crisis and the self-reinforcing pattern it creates as a burden spiral. The formal apparatus of oversight remains intact, but its capacity to sustain interpretive trust erodes.

This book argued that addressing the crisis requires a representational shift, not incremental process improvement. The necessary techniques largely exist. Descriptive workflow languages have matured in bioinformatics and are beginning to spread into broader data engineering. Domain-specific languages for data modelling can express transformation logic in terms that are both machine-executable and human-inspectable. Provenance capture is a recognised concern in research data management and platform governance. What has been missing is the integration of these elements into a coherent method: transformation-level provenance, automatically captured through a data modelling DSL, structured for query and comparison, portable across systems and abstract enough to support external predicates that encode recurring compliance and quality expectations. We termed this actionable provenance and showed how it provides the substrate for a narrow, data-centric form of compliance-as-code. This aligns with broader policy recognition that governance must become more computable if it is to remain effective at scale.

Parts I and III developed the conceptual architecture: complete provenance as a technical requirement, delegated understanding as the function regulation performs, operational, epistemic and interpretive trust as the dimensions at stake, and the burden

M. Bouzinier et al., *Research Data that Can Be Trusted*, SpringerBriefs in Computer Science, https://doi.org/10.1007/978-3-032-21032-6

spiral as the structural problem that current practice cannot resolve. Parts II and IV confirmed that the approach is realisable. The Medicare claims case study demonstrated transformation-level lineage under realistic constraints. The taxonomy of transformations and validation operators provided the semantic vocabulary on which portable predicates depend.

The claim is limited but consequential. Transformation-level provenance does not automate governance or encode whole legal regimes. It makes part of assurance more continuous and less episodic by enabling structured checks over recorded behaviour. Benefits depend on adoption discipline: coverage must prioritise transformations that materially affect validity and risk, semantics must be governed and predicates must be curated rather than allowed to sprawl.

The next step is convergence on shared semantic baselines and practical interfaces through which workflow engines, data platforms and governance processes can exchange computable process evidence. If that convergence occurs, provenance can function as a common evidentiary layer across research, institutional governance and regulatory review, sustaining interpretive trust where human-bounded inspection alone no longer suffices.

Appendix A
Syntax of YAML-Based Dorieh Data Modeling Language

Core Data Modeling Language

The Dorieh core data modeling language describes database objects such as tables, relationships between them (e.g., foreign keys), indices and conventions that govern things like naming and roles of specific columns.

We assume that a model is defined for a specific knowledge domain. Across domains, data can be linked based on column-naming conventions. For instance, a column named 'zipcode' always represents a US ZIP code, regardless of domain and thus can be used for linkages and aggregations.

This section describes the following language constructs:

- Domain
- Table
  - Create statement
  - Invalid record handling
- Column
  - Source
  - Index
  - Generated columns
  - Computed columns
  - File columns
  - Record columns
  - Transposing columns
  - Wildcards
- Multi-column indices
- Generation of the database schema (DDL)
- Indexing policies
- Linking with nomenclature

M. Bouzinier et al., *Research Data that Can Be Trusted*,
SpringerBriefs in Computer Science, https://doi.org/10.1007/978-3-032-21032-6

Domain

Handling domains is implemented by the Domain class.

For each domain, its data model is defined by a YAML file in the src/yml directory.

Each model is represented by a "forest": a set of tree-like structures of tables. It can contain one or several root tables.

The domain must be the first entry in the YAML file, for example:

```
my_domain:
```

The following parameters can be defined for domain:

Parameter	Required?	Description
schema	yes	Database schema, in which all tables are generated
schema.audit	no	Database schema for tables containing audit logs of data ingestion, including corrupted, duplicate and inconsistent records
index	no	Default indexing policy for this domain. This policy is used for tables that do not define their own indexing policy
tables	yes	list of table definitions
description	no	description of this domain to be included in auto-generated documentation
reference	no	URL with external documentation
header	no	Boolean value, passed to CSV loader. Describes input source rather than data model itself
quoting	no	One of the following values: QUOTE_MINIMAL (or MINIMAL), QUOTE_ALL (or ALL), QUOTE_NONNUMERIC (or NONNUMERIC), QUOTE_NONE (or NONE), passed to CSV loader. Describes input source rather than data model itself. Numeric values are accepted for compatibility (QUOTE_MINIMAL = 0, QUOTE_ALL = 1, QUOTE_NONNUMERIC = 2, QUOTE_NONE = 3)

Table

The following parameters can be defined for a table:

Parameter	Required?	Description
type	no	view/table
hard_linked	no	Denotes that the table is an integral part of parent table rather than a separate table with a many-to-one relationship to the parent table
columns	yes	list of column definitions
indices or indexes	yes	dictionary of multi-column indices
primary_key	yes	list of column names included in the table primary key

(continued)

(continued)

Parameter	Required?	Description
children	no	list of table definitions for child tables of this table
description	no	description of this table to be included in auto-generated documentation
reference	no	URL with external documentation
invalid.records	no	action to be performed upon encountering an invalid record (corrupted, incomplete, duplicate, etc.)
create	no	If the table or view should be created from existing database objects, see detailed description

Create statement

Describes how a table or a view should be created.

Parameter	Required?	Description
type	no	view / table
select	no	columns to put in SELECT clause of CREATE statement
from	no	What to put into FROM clause
group by	no	What to put into GROUP BY clause
populate	no, default is True	If false, a condition that can never be satisfied is added as a WHERE clause, so an empty table is created, which can be populated later. This is mostly used when additional triggers are needed for the population process

Invalid record

By default, an exception is raised if an invalid record is encountered during data ingestion. However, it is possible to override this behaviour by instructing the data loader to either ignore such records or put them in a special audit table.

Parameter	Required?	Description
action	yes	Action to be performed: INSERT or IGNORE
target	yes/no	For action INSERT - a target table
description	no	description to be included in auto-generated documentation
reference	no	URL with external documentation

Column

Parameter	Required?	Description
type	yes	Database type
source	no	source of the data
requires	no	List of tables and views required to compute this column. Should be used if source is a SQL statement referencing other tables
index	no	Override default to build an index based on this column. Possible values: true/false/dictionary. See index
description	no	description of this column to be included in auto-generated documentation
reference	no	URL with external documentation

Besides "normal" columns, when the value is directly taken from a column in a tabular input source, there are three types of special columns:

- Computed columns
- Generated columns
- Transposed columns (i.e., when multiple columns of a single record are converted to multiple records)

Special columns must have their source defined. If a column name in input source is different from a column name in the database, such column must also define source.

Source

Source must be defined for special columns and for columns whose name in the database differs from the name in the input source.

Parameter	Required?	Description
column name	no	A column name in the incoming tabular data
type	no	Types: generated, multi_column, range, compute, file
range	no	
code	no	Code for generated and computed columns
columns	no	
parameters	no	

Index

The value for index key can be a simple boolean true or false. If additional parameters are required, the value can be a dictionary with the following keys. For the explanation of options like *using* or *include*, see PostgreSQL Documentation.

Parameter	Required?	Description
name	no	A custom index name, if omitted the name will be generated
using	no	The indexing method, the default is BTREE
include	no	Additional columns to include with index
required_before_loading_data	no	Adding this key tells the generator that this index must be created before the table is populated. Otherwise, to improve performance, indices might be created after a table is populated with all data

Generated columns

Generated columns are columns that are not present in the source (e.g. CSV or FST file) but whose value is automatically computed using other columns values, or another deterministic expression **inside the database**.

From PostgreSQL Documentation:

> Theoretically, generated columns are for columns what a view is for tables. There are two kinds of generated columns: stored and virtual. A stored generated column is computed when it is written (inserted or updated) and occupies storage as if it were a normal column. A virtual generated column occupies no storage and is computed when it is read. Thus, a virtual generated column is similar to a view and a stored generated column is similar to a materialized view (except that it is always updated automatically).
>
> However, **PostgreSQL currently implements only STORED generated columns**.

Computed columns

Computed columns are columns that are not present in the source (e.g. CSV or FST file) but whose value is computed using provided Python code by the Universal Database Loader. They use the values of other columns in the same record and can call out to standard Python functions.

The columns used for computation are listed in either columns or parameters sections. Column names are names of the original columns in the data file. To reference columns in the database use parameters. Referenced them by a number in curly brackets in the compute code.

Here is an example of a computed column:

```
- admission_date:
    type: "DATE"
    source:
        type: "compute"
        columns:
            - "ADMSN_DT"
        code: "datetime.strptime({1}, '%Y%m%d').date()"
```

Here, in the code, the pattern {1} is replaced with the name of the first (and only) column in the list: ADMSN_DT.

Another example, using database columns:

```
- fips5:
    source:
      type: "compute"
      parameters:
        - state
        - residence_county
      code: "fips_dict[{1}] * 1000 + int({2})"
```

Here, {1} references the value that would be inserted into the table column state and {2} references the value that would be inserted into the table column residence_county.

File columns

File columns are of type file. They store the name of the file, from which the data has been ingested.

Record columns

Record columns are of type record. They store the sequential index of the record (line number) in the file, from which the data has been ingested.

Transposing columns

Columns can be exploded (unnested) or collapsed.

Exploding is useful, for example, when there is a separate column for each month. The easiest way to do this is to combine these monthly columns into an array and then use the PostgreSQL unnest function.

Wildcards

To make it easier to work with similarly named columns, Dorieh supports wildcards. Wildcard expression starts with $ followed by a single letter. Values are provided in square brackets that follow a wildcard.

Example:

```
- diag[$n=1:25]:
    type: varchar
    optional: true
    source:

      - dgnscd$n
```

Will be expanded to 25 columns named diag1, diag2 ,..., diag25.

Multi-column indices

Multi-column indices of a table are defined in the indices section (spelling indexes is also acceptable). This is a dictionary with an index name as a key and its definition as the value. At the very minimum, the definition should include the list of the columns to be used in the index.

Index definition can also include index type (e.g. btree, hash, etc.) and data to be included with the index.

Parameter	Required?	Description
columns	yes	A list of columns to include in the index
using	no	The indexing method, the default is BTREE
include	no	Additional columns to include with index
unique	no	Specifies that the index defines a unique constraint

Example:

```
indices:
  adm_ys_idx:
    columns:
      - state
      - year
  adm_ys_iso_idx:
    columns:
      - state_iso
      - year
    include:
      - bene
```

Generation of the database schema (DDL)

From a domain YAML file, the database schema is generated in the form of the PostgreSQL dialect of DDL.

The main class responsible for the generation of DDL is Domain.

Indexing policies

- **explicit**. Indices are only created for columns that define an index
- **all** Indices are created for all columns
- **selected** Indices are created only for columns matching certain pattern (defined in index_columns variable of model) module
- **unless excluded** Indices are created for all columns not explicitly excluded

Linking with nomenclature

US States

The database includes a table with codes for US states. It is taken from:

https://www.nrcs.usda.gov/wps/portal/nrcs/detail/national/technical/nra/nri/results/?cid=nrcs143_013696

The data lives locally in fips.py.

County codes:

https://www.nber.org/research/data/ssa-federal-information-processing-series-fips-state-and-county-crosswalk

Data Modeling Language Extensions

These extensions are implemented by Dorieh for practical purposes, however, they are of an ad hoc nature and have not been formally incorporated into the language.

The following constructs are described here:

- Combining data from different tables (approximate **union** operation)
- Casting data types
- Validating consistency of data across tables

Combining Multiple Sources and Optional Columns

Source can be an array of columns rather than one column.

The following block will define a column named ssa3. The tool will look for columns named either cnty_cd, or bene_county_cd, or ssa_county to map to the new ssa3 column. If neither of these three columns is found, a new column will be created and filled with NULL values.

Without optional: true, if an appropriate source column is not found, an exception will be raised.

Example:

```
- ssa3:
    optional: true
    description: Social Security Administration (SSA) three digit code for
county
    reference: https://www.nber.org/research/data/ssa-federal-information-
processing-series-fips-state-and-county-crosswalk
    source:
      - cnty_cd
      - bene_county_cd
      - ssa_county
```

Exclude

Using exclude in a create block can exclude certain tables matching a pattern from the federated view.

The following example creates a view by combining all tables matching either cms.mbsf_ab* or cms.mcr_bene_* pattern, but excluding the table named mbsf_ab_2015:

```
ps:
  create:
    type: view
    from:

      - cms.mbsf_ab*
      - cms.mcr_bene_*
    exclude:
      - mbsf_ab_2015
```

Cast

It is possible to define custom casts from one type to another. When tables to be combined into a single view have columns containing corresponding data but of different types, it is possible to cast all of them to the same type.

In the following example:

```
- dob:
    type: date
    cast:
      "character varying": "public.parse_date({column_name})"
      numeric: "to_date(to_char({column_name}, '00000000'), 'YYYYMMDD')"
      *: {column_name}::DATE
```

- If a source column is of type DATE, it will be left as-is
- If the source column is of numeric type, the code to_date (to_char({column_name}, '00000000'), 'YYYYMMDD') will be used to transform the source value
- If the source column has type character varying, then the function public.parse_date will be called to transform the value
- For all other types a simple PostgreSQL cast will be attempted

Appendix B
Towards Better Expressiveness: From YAML to Groovy and Nextflow

Motivation

While our YAML-based DSL is sufficiently powerful to express the data transformations discussed in this book, it has several downsides:

1. **Modularity**. Modularity drastically improves both readability and maintainability of code and facilitates distributed development and collaboration. While some support for modular YAML scripts exists in many tools (e.g., Home Assistant, Bitrise, RPM), it is not standardized. The lack of modularity leads to over-indentation and other readability problems. Navigating large YAML files is challenging.
2. **Integration with workflow languages**. Among popular workflow languages, only CWL uses YAML syntax. However, because YAML lacks standardized modularity, it does not easily accommodate integration of a descriptive data-transformation sublanguage.
3. **Expressiveness for non-technical users**. YAML syntax is quite rigid, and large YAML scripts are difficult to read for less technical subject-matter experts.

Many of these issues can be alleviated by using a different base toolkit for the DSL. In particular, Apache Groovy looks attractive. Groovy provides ideal conditions for creating DSLs due to features such as closures, optional parentheses and dots and builder syntax. These features allow developers to define custom control structures and fluent APIs.

Groovy DSLs are ultimately syntactic sugar on top of a standard API (often a Java API). Groovy code is parsed and executed, usually with a delegate object that implements the underlying logic. This makes it possible for scripts to look less like traditional code and more like a notation customized for subject-matter experts in the target domain. Consequently, we can tailor Groovy dialects specifically for health-data practitioners and policy makers.

M. Bouzinier et al., *Research Data that Can Be Trusted*, SpringerBriefs in Computer Science, https://doi.org/10.1007/978-3-032-21032-6

Similarly to how CWL uses YAML syntax, Nextflow uses Groovy. However, because Groovy has built-in support for modularity, integration between a Groovy-based data-transformation DSL and Nextflow can be seamless.

In Dorieh, we have developed a prototype Groovy parser that can translate the example below into the currently implemented YAML dialect. The parser is available in our GitHub repository.

Example: DSL for Healthcare IT Practitioners

The following example illustrates how a Groovy-based DSL can express the same concepts as our YAML-based DSL, but in a form that is often more readable for healthcare IT practitioners. Note how it describes tables, transformations and aggregation logic in a declarative, domain-specific style.

```
table ps {
 type = 'view'
 union of {
   - 'cms.mbsf_ab*'

   - 'cms.mcr_bene_*'
 }

 columns {
   bene_id ('STRING')

   year {
     type = 'INT'
     isomorphic_transformation of ("year")
     sql =
     '''
     CASE
       WHEN "year"::int < 20 THEN (2000 + "year"::int)
       WHEN (20 < "year"::int AND "year"::int < 100) THEN (1900 + "year"::int)
       WHEN "year" IS NULL THEN 2000 ELSE "year"::int
     END
     '''
   }

   dob {
     type = "DATE"
     description = """
     Date of birth
     """
     isomorphic_transformation of (
             dob,
             bene_dob,
             bene_birth_dt
     )
```

```
      cast (
              "character varying": "public.parse_date({column_name})",
              "numeric": "to_date(to_char({column_name}, '00000000'), 'YYYYMMDD')"
)
    }
  }
}

table beneficiaries {
 aggregation of ( "ps" )
 on (bene_id)
 reconcile {
   dob {
     pick "max" over "min"
     record "count distinct"
   }
   dod {
     pick "min" over "max"
     record ("count distinct")
   }
 }

   aggregate {
     first_enrollment_year = MIN(year)

     last_enrollment_year = MAX (year)
     all_enrollment_years = "ARRAY_AGG(DISTINCT year ORDER BY year)"
   }
  }

  domain Medicare {
   name 'medicare'
   schema = 'medicare'
   auditSchema = 'medicare_audit'
   quoting = '3'
   indexingPolicy = 'unless excluded'

   tables {
     ps
     beneficiaries
   }
  }


  workflow {
   domain "Medicare"
   build "beneficiaries"
  }
```

Example: DSL for Policy Makers and Governance Experts

The next, more ambitious example sketches a Groovy dialect aimed at health-data policy makers and governance experts. The goal is to express legal and regulatory constraints (EHDS, GDPR) directly in the data-transformation specification, in a way that remains readable for non-technical stakeholders.

```
// European Health Data Space (EHDS) Compliance
transform patient_outcomes {
  from: bronze.clinical_records
  ehds_compliance: {
    // EHDS Article 33: Purpose limitation for secondary use
    purpose_of_use: {
      category: "scientific_research"
      specific_purpose: "cardiovascular_outcomes_study"
      ethics_approval: "ETH-2024-0142"
      lawful_basis: "public_interest_research"
    }
    // EHDS Article 34: Data categories for secondary use
    permitted_categories: [
      "diagnosis_codes",       // ICD-10
      "procedure_codes",       // SNOMED-CT
      "lab_results",          // LOINC codes only
      "medications",          // ATC classification
      "demographics"          // age, gender, region only
    ]
    // EHDS Article 44: Health data access bodies requirements
    access_environment: {
      secure_processing: true
      data_localization: "EU"
      cross_border_transfer: false
    }
    // GDPR Article 89: Safeguards for research
    safeguards: {
      pseudonymization: true
      encryption_at_rest: "AES-256"
      access_logging: "comprehensive"
    }
  }
  pseudonymization_rules: {
    patient_id → hash(salt: project_specific)
    birth_date → age_at_event
    admission_date → relative_timeline(index_date: "diagnosis")
    hospital_id → region_category
    treating_physician → "removed"
  }
```

```
  quality_predicates: [
    // Statistical disclosure control
    assert_k_anonymity(k: 5, quasi_identifiers: ["age", "gender",
"region"]),
    assert_l_diversity(l: 3, sensitive: "primary_diagnosis"),
    // Data quality
    assert_completeness(critical_fields: ["diagnosis", "outcome"],
threshold: 0.95),
    assert_temporal_consistency(date_fields: ["admission", "discharge",
"procedure"]),
    // Consent and purpose
    assert_valid_consent(type: "broad_consent_research"),
    assert_purpose_compatibility(declared: "cardiovascular", used_for:
"cardiovascular")
  ]
  to: silver.cardiovascular_cohort
  provenance_capture: {
    transformation_graph: true,
    compliance_attestation: generate_signed(),
    validation_report: comprehensive,
    retention_period: "10_years"  // EHDS audit requirement
  }
}
```

Glossary of Terms

Actionable provenance A form of provenance that records data transformations in a structured, machine-interpretable way so that they can be automatically queried and checked against external rules (e.g., regulatory or quality constraints).

Admission (inpatient admission) A hospitalization episode, typically represented as a record in claims data (e.g., MEDPAR), with fields such as admission and discharge dates, diagnoses and facility information.

Admissions table A harmonized, silver-layer dataset that normalizes and enriches inpatient admissions across years and raw files, often adding standardized dates, locations, diagnosis arrays and validation flags.

Aggregation (simple aggregation) A transformation that combines multiple input values into a single value (e.g., MIN, MAX, COUNT, AVG, STRING_AGG), inherently non-reversible because it summarizes detailed data.

Approximation operator (approximation) A transformation that infers or estimates missing or ambiguous values (e.g., inferring a county FIPS code from a ZIP code). It may produce plausible but not guaranteed-correct values and is not reversible.

Array flattening/unnesting Flattening aggregates multiple values into a single array; unnesting does the reverse by expanding array elements into multiple rows. Unlike many aggregations, flattening + unnesting can be reversible.

Artificial Intelligence (AI) Computational methods, often based on machine learning, that learn patterns from data to perform tasks such as prediction, classification, or decision support.

AI Act (European Union Artificial Intelligence Act) The EU's horizontal regulation for AI systems, classifying certain systems (including many healthcare applications) as "high-risk" and imposing requirements for dataset governance, documentation, risk management and transparency.

Beneficiaries table A silver-layer table in the Medicare pipeline that aggregates enrollment information to one record per beneficiary, applying disambiguation rules for attributes such as date of birth, date of death, race and sex and recording ambiguity explicitly.

M. Bouzinier et al., *Research Data that Can Be Trusted*, SpringerBriefs in Computer Science, https://doi.org/10.1007/978-3-032-21032-6

Bronze/Silver/Gold layers (Medallion Architecture) A multi-tiered data architecture:

- **Bronze**: as-ingested or minimally processed data (close to raw).
- **Silver**: cleaned, harmonized and enriched data suitable for general analytics.
- **Gold**: aggregated, analysis- or ML-ready datasets tailored to specific questions or consumers.

Burden spiral (volume crisis) A systemic dynamic where growing regulatory and governance demands require more documentation than human reviewers can realistically interpret, leading to ever-increasing reporting without proportional gains in understanding or trust.

Cell-level lineage Provenance that traces the origin and transformations of individual cell values (intersection of row and column), rather than only entire columns or tables.

Clinical decision support (CDS) Systems or tools that use data and models to assist clinicians in diagnosis, risk prediction, or treatment decisions, often powered by ML/AI.

Cohort restriction A transformation that filters records to define a study or training population according to inclusion and exclusion criteria.

Column-level lineage Provenance that records how each output column is derived from upstream columns across datasets and transformations.

Compliance-as-code (data-centric sense) The practice of expressing selected regulatory or governance conditions as executable rules (predicates) over structured provenance, so that conformance can be checked automatically.

Computable trust An approach to trust where part of the evidentiary work (e.g., checking whether pipelines respect certain constraints) can be performed automatically by evaluating rules over structured provenance, with humans interpreting the results.

Common Workflow Language (CWL) A descriptive workflow definition language designed to specify portable, reproducible computational pipelines by declaring tools, inputs, outputs and DAG topology.

Croissant-RAI A machine-readable dataset documentation format proposed for Responsible AI, defining structured metadata fields (e.g., for preprocessing, missing data, annotation) that can be aligned with provenance-oriented DSLs.

CWL-Airflow An integration that translates CWL workflow descriptions into Airflow DAGs, allowing CWL workflows to run within Apache Airflow.

Data dictionary Structured documentation describing datasets, tables and fields (including types, meanings, units and derivations). In Dorieh, data dictionaries are generated automatically from the DSL and used with lineage diagrams.

Data flow/data pipeline A sequence of steps that extract, transform and load data from raw sources to analytic or ML-ready outputs, typically represented as a Directed Acyclic Graph (DAG).

Data governance The set of policies, processes and controls that determine how data are collected, transformed, accessed and used, especially regarding quality, privacy, ethics and regulatory compliance.

Data lineage A record of where data come from and how they move through transformations over time; often represented as a graph linking source datasets, steps and outputs.

Data modeling DSL (Domain-Specific Language) A specialized, descriptive language used in this book to define dataset structures and transformations (e.g., field construction operators, validation rules) in a human- and machine-readable way, distinct from general-purpose programming.

Data preparation (data preprocessing) All transformations applied to raw data before analysis or model training, including normalization, harmonization, cleansing, aggregation and feature construction.

Data provenance The complete, structured history of data, including origins, collection context, transformations, assumptions and validation steps; the central concept of the book.

Data quality The degree to which data are accurate, complete, consistent, timely and fit for their intended use, often assessed via validation checks and QC aggregates.

Data warehouse A centralized repository optimized for analytical queries, storing structured data (often in normalized or star schemas) that feed research, reporting and feature stores .

Dataset operator A node in a dataflow DAG that takes one or more input datasets and produces one or more output datasets, defined as a union of independent field construction operators and assumed to operate on immutable inputs.

Decision support system A system that uses data and models to support operational or clinical decisions, often in real time, such as risk scores or alerting tools.

Descriptive dataflow operator A data transformation operator defined in a descriptive DSL that states what the transformation does (semantically) rather than prescribing how to implement it procedurally, enabling compilation to different backends and rich provenance.

Descriptive workflow language A workflow language (e.g., CWL, Nextflow, Snakemake, WDL) that focuses on declaratively describing pipeline steps, inputs/outputs and dependencies, leaving execution details to specific engines.

Directed Acyclic Graph (DAG) A graph structure with directed edges and no cycles; used to represent workflow topology, where nodes are tasks/operators and edges represent data or dependency relationships.

Dorieh Data Platform An Apache-licensed, open-source data platform developed at Harvard that implements the DSL concepts in this book, combining CWL for workflow topology with a YAML-based data modeling DSL, PostgreSQL backend and lineage/documentation tools.

DSL (Domain-Specific Language) A programming or specification language tailored to a particular domain. In this book, DSLs are used to describe data transformations, datasets and validation rules in a form suitable for provenance capture.

EHDS (European Health Data Space) An EU regulatory and infrastructural initiative to enable secure, governed primary and secondary use of health data across Member States, including requirements for data quality, labelling and access bodies.

Electronic Health Record (EHR) A longitudinal digital record of a patient's clinical encounters, diagnoses, procedures, medications, etc., typically used as a primary data source for secondary analyses.

ELT (Extract-Load-Transform) A variant of ETL where raw data are loaded into a storage system first and then transformed within that system.

Epistemic trust Trust in the correctness and usefulness of the results or conclusions produced by a system (e.g., model predictions or study findings), dependent on operational and interpretive trust.

ETL (Extract-Transform-Load) A pattern for data pipelines in which source data are extracted, transformed and then loaded into a target system such as a data warehouse.

Feature store A system that manages, documents and serves reusable ML features, ensuring that training and inference see consistent feature definitions and (in this book's view) should be backed by robust provenance and data dictionaries.

Federated admissions view A harmonized silver-layer view that unifies inpatient admission records from multiple year- or format-specific raw tables into a single schema.

Federated patient summary (ps) view A harmonized silver -layer view that unifies beneficiary/enrollment information from multiple MBSF -like tables into a single schema with standardized fields.

FILE directive A DSL directive that instructs ingestion tools to add a field capturing the original file name or URI for each ingested record, supporting row-level lineage.

FIPS code (Federal Information Processing Standards code) Standardized numeric codes used to identify US states and counties, frequently used for geographic rollups and harmonization.

Flattening (array aggregation) Turning multiple values into a single array value (e.g., aggregating diagnosis columns into an array), which can later be unnested back into multiple rows.

Gold layer The medallion layer containing analytic- or ML-ready tables and materialized views, such as state-level climate aggregates or QC tables, derived exclusively from Silver.

Governance diversity The condition in which multiple overlapping regulatory and policy frameworks (e.g., data protection, sectoral rules, ethics, AI regulations) impose different expectations on the same data pipelines.

Harmonization Transforming semantically similar but structurally or format-wise different data (e.g., from different years or systems) into a consistent schema and coding system.

HealthDCAT-AP An application profile extending DCAT-AP for health datasets, used to publish and describe health data in a machine-readable way and potentially aligned with provenance-oriented documentation.

HIPAA (Health Insurance Portability and Accountability Act) A US law that, among other things, regulates the privacy and security of protected health information (PHI), influencing requirements for de-identification and secure processing.

HL7 FHIR (Fast Healthcare Interoperability Resources) A standard for structuring and exchanging healthcare data, used as one of several clinical data models mentioned in the book.

HPO (Human Phenotype Ontology) An ontology of standardized terms describing human phenotypic abnormalities, used for specialized diagnostic or research coding.

HyperLogLog (HLL) A probabilistic algorithm for approximate counting of distinct elements (e.g., distinct beneficiaries), used as a custom aggregation to support scalable QC metrics.

ICD (International Classification of Diseases) A standard medical classification for diagnoses, used extensively in claims and clinical data (e.g., ICD -9, ICD -10), often mapped to higher-level categories (e.g., Charlson Comorbidity Index).

Idempotency (of operators) The property that re-applying an operator multiple times has the same effect as applying it just once, preventing duplicate or unintended side effects.

Interpretive trust Trust that arises from being able to understand and trace what was done to data—i.e., from transparent, inspectable transformations and provenance, rather than just secure environments or validated outcomes.

Isomorphic transformation A reversible transformation where each output value uniquely corresponds to an input value (e.g., changing date formats, unit conversions), preserving information.

Journaling (of invalid records) The practice of storing records that fail validation in a dedicated audit table, along with failure reasons and provenance, instead of silently dropping them or aborting processing.

Lakehouse/Delta Live Tables (conceptual relation) A modern architectural pattern (popularized by Databricks) that unifies data warehousing and data lakes, often using medallion layering and table-as-code concepts analogous to Dorieh domains and dataset operators.

Lineage graph (data lineage graph) A graphical representation of how datasets and fields are derived from upstream sources and transformations, typically at table- or column-level in Dorieh.

Master Beneficiary Summary File (MBSF) A CMS file type containing annual "master" records of Medicare beneficiaries, including demographic and enrollment information, used as key input in the Medicare pipeline.

Medallion Architecture A layered data architecture pattern with Bronze, Silver and Gold stages, emphasizing progressive refinement of data and clear lineage across stages.

Medicare claims US health insurance claims for Medicare beneficiaries, including beneficiary summaries (MBSF) and inpatient admission files (e.g., MEDPAR), used as a central case study for provenance-aware pipelines.

MEDPAR (Medicare Provider Analysis and Review) A CMS file containing inpatient claim records for Medicare beneficiaries, including admission/discharge dates and diagnoses.

Missing data imputation The process of filling in missing values using statistical or rule-based methods; in this book is often treated as an approximation step to be explicitly recorded in provenance.

Non-isomorphic transformation A transformation that loses information, so that the original input cannot be fully reconstructed from the output (e.g., hashing identifiers, truncating strings, many rollups).

Normalization (in this taxonomy) Transforming values to a canonical representation (e.g., consistent date format, all lower-case strings, temperature to Kelvin). Although some technical information may be lost, the goal is not to coarsen semantics but to standardize representation.

OMOP Common Data Model (OMOP CDM) A widely used observational health data model that standardizes the structure and content of clinical data for multi-site research and analytics.

Operational trust Trust in the security and reliability of the technical environment (e.g., access controls, encryption, audit logs), ensuring that data are protected and systems behave as expected at an infrastructural level.

Pandas A popular Python data analysis library, mentioned as an in-memory tool that does not by itself provide scalable provenance tracking.

Personally identifiable information (PII) Information that can be used to identify an individual, either directly or in combination with other data; in healthcare often subject to strict regulatory protections.

PHI (Protected Health Information) A subset of health-related PII covered by HIPAA, including identifiers tied to medical information, requiring stringent safeguards.

Predicate over provenance An executable rule or query that inspects structured provenance (e.g., checking imputation rates, exclusion patterns, or use of sensitive fields) to determine whether certain constraints are satisfied.

Primary key/foreign key A primary key uniquely identifies records in a table; a foreign key references records in another table. Key integrity is a major target of validation checks.

Provenance, transformation-level Provenance that records data-processing events (transformations and their parameters) at the level of individual operators, rather than only dataset-level inputs and outputs.

Pseudonymization The replacement of direct identifiers with pseudonyms (e.g., salted hashes), allowing linkage across datasets without exposing raw identifiers; should be recorded explicitly in provenance.

QC (Quality Control) table A Gold-layer table that aggregates measures of data quality and validation outcomes (e.g., counts of ambiguous DOBs, proportions of invalid admissions) by year, geography, or other dimensions.

Record-level validation Validation checks applied to individual records (e.g., primary key completeness, date plausibility), often determining whether a record is accepted, rejected, or journaled.

RECORD directive A DSL directive that adds a per-record index (line number in the source file), enabling precise row-level lineage back to raw files.

ResDAC (Research Data Assistance Center) The CMS-affiliated organization that distributes Medicare data and documentation (e.g., fixed-width files and FTS documents) to approved researchers.

Resilient Distributed Dataset (RDD) An abstraction in Apache Spark for fault-tolerant, distributed collections of data, enabling large-scale transformations.

Rollup A many-to-one transformation that aggregates or generalizes detailed values into higher-level categories (e.g., county to state, ICD codes to comorbidity index), reducing granularity and losing some information.

Row-level lineage Provenance that tracks how a particular record in an output dataset relates to specific records in source datasets, often anchored by file name (FILE) and record index (RECORD).

Secure Processing Environment/Trusted Research Environment (TRE) A controlled infrastructure where sensitive data (e.g., health or claims data) are hosted and accessed under strict governance, security and auditing conditions.

SHAP (SHapley Additive exPlanations) A method based on Shapley values from cooperative game theory used to explain individual model predictions; mentioned as complementary to provenance for understanding AI behaviour.

Silver layer The medallion layer that contains cleaned, harmonized and enriched tables and views (e.g., ps, beneficiaries, enrollments, admissions), serving as the basis for Gold aggregates.

Snakemake/Nextflow/WDL Popular descriptive workflow languages/frameworks that define and execute pipelines via DAGs, focusing on the what of pipeline topology rather than imperative control flow.

Source dataset/raw data Original data as delivered by producers (e.g., ResDAC fixed-width files), before harmonization, normalization, or cleansing.

Structured documentation Machine-and human-readable descriptions (e.g., DSL definitions, Croissant-RAI metadata, data dictionaries) that systematically capture dataset and transformation properties.

Table-level lineage A view of lineage where nodes are tables or views and edges connect them according to derivation relationships (e.g., Bronze → Silver → Gold).

TEHDAS (Towards European Health Data Space) EU joint actions that develop infrastructure, governance and quality frameworks to support the EHDS, including concepts such as dataset labelling.

Transformation (data transformation) Any operation that changes the content, structure, or representation of data, including single-value functions, aggregations, rollups, unions, approximations and reshaping.

Trusted Research Environment (TRE) See Secure Processing Environment.

Union transformation A transformation that combines records from multiple datasets (often spanning years or sources) into a single unified dataset, handling field alignment and type casting as needed.

Validation (of data) A broad term in the book encompassing: • Data quality validation: checking that raw or intermediate data satisfy basic constraints (e.g., ranges, formats, key integrity). • Validation of algorithms: checking that transformations or algorithms behave as specified (e.g., via test cases or lineage-based spot checks). • Validation of constraints: checking that workflows comply with higher-level requirements (e.g., population coverage, exclusion rules), possibly using provenance without direct access to data.

Volume crisis See Burden spiral.

WDL (Workflow Definition Language) A descriptive language for specifying computational workflows, similar in spirit to CWL and Nextflow.

Workflow engine/orchestrator Software that executes workflow definitions (e.g., Airflow, Nextflow, CWL runners), managing task scheduling, dependencies and resource allocation.

YAML-based DSL The initial implementation of DSL using YAML syntax.

ZCTA (ZIP Code Tabulation Area) A Census-defined geographic approximation of US ZIP Code service areas, used in the book's climate example for aggregating gridded data to postal regions.

Index

M. Bouzinier et al., *Research Data that Can Be Trusted*, SpringerBriefs in Computer Science, https://doi.org/10.1007/978-3-032-21032-6

W

Y

Z

The manufacturer's authorised representative in the EU is Springer Nature Customer Service Centre GmbH, Europaplatz 3, 69115 Heidelberg, Germany. If you have any concerns regarding our products, please contact ProductSafety@springernature.com

Printed and bound by CPI Group (UK) Ltd, Croydon, CR0 4YY
07/07/2026
02160920-0002